Poker Isometrics

and Poker Fitness

By Anton Drake

A Puragreen Productions LLC Publication

ISBN 978-0-9831502-0-6

Disclaimer

This book is intended for educational purposes only. The information, techniques, ideas and suggestions in this book are not intended as a substitute for professional medical advice. Always consult your physician or health care professional before performing any new exercise or fitness routine. The information on diet and nutritional supplements in this book is provided for educational purposes only, and is not intended to diagnose or treat any medical disorder. You are advised to consult with your physician before making any changes to your diet or taking any nutritional supplements.

Any application of the techniques, ideas, and suggestions in this book is at the reader's sole discretion and risk. Some of the exercises described in this book may be too strenuous for some people, and the reader should consult their health practitioner before engaging in them. The editors, authors and or publishers of this book make no warranty of any kind about the contents of this book or any of the information contained in it. Neither the author nor the publisher shall be liable or responsible for any injury, damage or loss allegedly arising, either directly or indirectly, from any of the information, techniques or suggestions contained within this book. Isometrics and other forms of exercise can be dangerous if performed improperly, especially if performed without proper pre-exercise medical evaluation, competent instruction and personal supervision from a qualified fitness professional and your physician. Readers are advised to consult with their physician or a qualified health care professional before beginning this program.

Contents

Introduction

Poker takes a physical toll

As a poker player, one thing you're very likely to become aware of sooner or later is that playing poker takes a physical toll on your body. The energy, or "juice", that drives poker players through long sessions at the tables is generated by intense thought and concentration, coupled with risk, competition, adrenaline, emotions and *action*. At the same time, to be a good poker player you must be able to control yourself—which is not always easy. When you're sitting at a poker table, sometimes for 10 or 12 hours or more, your body is basically *parked*. The only exercise you're likely to get during a poker game is from riffling your chips or walking to the bathroom or the bar. On a Vegas trip it's easy to find yourself on a schedule of playing poker, eating, sleeping, and playing more poker; playing until you're exhausted, then playing some more; fueling up on junk food and liquor, and sleeping fitfully for a few hours during the day, dreaming about poker hands. Sometimes it might feel as if you're immersed in one long, never-ending poker game, endlessly repeating the same pattern over and over again: waiting, folding, waiting, betting, raising, waiting, folding. At some point, you might start to feel that the game is literally playing itself, and that you are merely plugged into it, like a machine, reading hands and ranges, calculating odds, sizing bets, making strategy decisions and counting chips. However, while all this action is going on and your brain is so incredibly stimulated, your body is just *sitting* there, vegetating in an oftentimes smoke-filled casino. Occasionally you recharge by eating a hamburger or some pizza, and maybe have a beer. The bottom line is, if you play a lot of poker the sheer number of hours that you spend sitting on your butt will become a liability and an obstacle to your ultimate success in the game long term. There's just no way around this.

This simply can't be good for my body

Of course, if you have a lot of self-discipline and structure your poker sessions well, you can manage your day-to-day poker schedule intelligently—only playing for a set number of hours, and always quitting on time. You can insist on getting ample sleep, watch what you eat, and find the time each day to lift weights, go for a walk, get on the bike or go for a swim. But even for a player with a very reasonable and healthy poker schedule, the reality is all that sedentary (and sometimes stressful) time playing poker adds up, and over the course of a career it's a -EV factor for one's overall health and fitness. The sheer lack of physical activity and exercise that goes along with the life of a serious poker player may very well be one of the toughest opponents that any player faces in their career; and when combined with inconsistent sleep schedules, stress, drinking, overeating and even smoking, it may well prove dangerous to one's personal health and longevity. You may be very consistently profitable at your usual poker game; but we've all seen players who are obviously out of shape, and we've maybe wondered if that wasn't the inevitable destination for all of us eventually. The simple fact is that the more out of shape you are, the less energy, stamina, focus and well-being you'll possess; and if a player dies early from heart disease, stroke or any other disease linked to inactivity and stress, then the game is completely over.

Every serious poker player can remember mornings when they've walked out of a casino after an all-night session and thought to themselves "this can't be good for my body." Wobbling out of the casino into the light of a new day, with aching legs and a stiff, sore back, your brain hazy and wrung out, squinting through dry tired eyes, you've probably felt that eating a giant fast food burger for breakfast and falling asleep till the afternoon would be the healthiest thing you've done in days. Yet somewhere in the back of your mind is the question: "How can I possibly maintain this lifestyle for another twenty years?" And for all of us, it remains an open question whether we can win the long term battle between our body and the poker lifestyle.

Guess what: Poker Isometrics really works

What we will call Poker Isometrics, the systematic application of isometric muscle strengthening adapted for playing poker at the casino or on the Internet, can tremendously strengthen your body and improve your health, connecting you to your muscles and working them effectively during what are otherwise, for your body, wasted hours. And when I say tremendously, I do mean *tremendously*. As you begin to practice Poker Isometrics, you'll begin to develop a deep understanding of isometric muscle control and Core strength. You'll begin to find new ways to engage your muscles using isometrics—powerfully, invisibly and silently, and you'll start to love it, to become addicted to it, and to notice endless opportunities for using isometrics when your body would otherwise just be vegetating. While at first glance this concept may seem improbable or counter-intuitive, the fact of the matter is that Poker Isometrics *really works*. Consider a house cat: it sits or lies around the house 99% of the time; yet its muscles are toned and flexible, and its body literally shimmers with life and vitality. Even an ordinary house cat possesses an incredible mind-body connection, and can open its eyes from a relaxed nap and jump up onto a ten-foot wall an instant later. Cats instinctively flex and stretch their muscles, which keeps them fit and incredibly strong for their size, despite living indoors, or even in a cage.

The simple equation is this: isometric exercise really works; and many isometric exercises can be practiced very effectively while playing poker—silently, motionless and unnoticed. The concept of isometric exercise is well known: top athletes, bodybuilders, yogis and fighters have always used isometrics in one way or another. And sitting at the poker table can be an ideal setting for practicing many forms of isometric technique. For the poker player, one of the hidden advantages of practicing isometrics is that you'll have *many* hours of opportunity to practice, many hours where you already sitting down and completely absorbed in playing poker and not doing anything else—hours when you can easily multi-task and do isometrics. Someone who doesn't play poker will have to set aside specific blocks of time to practice isometrics, while the poker player can mix in isometric exercise as a stress reliever, a stimulant and a welcome diversion. As a poker player, you're already putting the time in sitting there; and even if you practice isometrics only 5% of that time, it can add up to significant practice, leading to rapid proficiency and mastery, which in turn leads to physical excellence. The fact that many of the isometric concepts you'll learn in this book can *best* be practiced from a seated position and, practiced correctly, don't require any outward bodily movement, can give the poker player an actual *advantage* in strengthening their body over a normal person. A poker player *will* put in the time, consistently, and the incredible effectiveness of the techniques *will* generate great results. You can practice Poker Isometrics *when* you want, for as *long* as you want, and it will always pay off:

1. Become physically stronger and improve your muscle tone
2. Reduce stress, and lower your blood pressure
3. Improve your mental focus and endurance
4. Lower your risk of heart attack and stroke
5. Strengthen and tighten your joints
6. Improve your posture and body alignment
7. Improve your circulation
8. Become more attractive, sexier and strengthen your sexual response
9. Stay off Tilt, and get un-Tilted when you need to
10. Reduce and conceal your involuntary poker tells effectively

You may or may not have heard of isometrics before; but the fact remains that various forms of isometric exercise have been known and practiced for thousands of years; modern science simply helps us to understand what isometrics is and why it works. But the ultimate knowledge exists within your own body. We've noted that the basic principles of isometrics can be seen in the way that a cat instinctively flexes and stretches its muscles; and these principles have been utilized and refined by some of the greatest yogis, martial artists, wrestlers, strongmen, bodybuilders and athletes who have ever lived. Once you begin to understand what isometrics is, you will automatically begin to improve your physical condition; and as your understanding of isometrics deepens, you will find new doors of physical strength and awareness opening for you. It is as if merely understanding the concept of isometrics will cause your muscles to start getting stronger.

Technique, insight and self-knowledge lead to *real* results

This book maps out the path of how to use isometrics at the poker table safely and effectively. This map consists of descriptions, photographs and diagrams explaining and demonstrating the positions and techniques, including a lot of very advanced insights and subtle adjustments. The idea is to help you "find" isometrics in your own body: the counter-tension and internal resistance of your own muscles working with each other, the push, pull and interconnectedness of your muscle groups, and your mental ability to control, isolate, flex and *use* that muscular counter-tension effectively to work your muscles intensely from a sitting, stationary position. Keep in mind that some of these concepts are subtle and deep and demand experience and practice; there is *always* more to learn about your own body, and the possibilities are endless. Understanding the mechanics of using your own body to generate isometric contractions is one thing, but experiencing the internal feelings and intuitions of your mind-body connection requires practice and deeper insight. I encourage you to innovate and experiment with variations, adjustments and combinations of techniques when you practice. If you read this book, you'll find that it will get you pointed in the right direction, and get you hot-wired and jump-started, awakening a new enthusiasm for physical excellence and physical fitness.

In addition to all of the Poker Isometrics theory and application, I've also included a few simple restorative techniques that you can do *away* from the poker table, at home or in your hotel room; these are deceptively simple and can really give your body a big boost recovering from stress and fatigue. I've also included chapters on diet, nutrition and supplements specifically for poker players. I'm a believer in good nutrition and nutritional supplements, and these chapters are loaded with some very high octane information on how to increase your energy, lower your risk of cardiovascular disease, and add years to your life. Good poker players always think in terms of value: take a moment to consider the value of every extra healthy year you can add to your life; and consider, also, the value of feeling better, stronger and more vital every day.

Isometric Theory

How do muscles work?

Muscles are made of fibers; when muscle fibers contract they shorten, which pulls on the skeleton and produces movement in the body. Muscles are attached to the skeleton with tendons and ligaments; muscular contraction creates pull, which translates into movement. Muscles in the body generally come in what can be called antagonistic pairs; an example of such a pair would be the muscles of the upper arm: the biceps and the triceps. Both the biceps and the triceps move the elbow joint: the contraction of the *biceps* bends the elbow, pulling the forearm toward the upper arm; while the contraction of the *triceps* on the back of the upper arm pulls the elbow straight. This natural muscular symmetry allows you to bend or straighten your elbow in various degrees, and to control its movement.

Origins of Isometrics

If we observe cats in the wild, we can see that they employ isometric principles naturally and instinctively. Anyone who's kept cats has seen them stretch themselves out and flex, the muscles of their body trembling with the force of it; likewise you've probably seen chimps at the zoo pushing and pulling and hanging on rocks and trees, their arms and backs flexed like woven steel. Yet you might not have guessed at the full extent of a chimp's actual strength: a 70-kilo chimp is easily *five times as strong* as a full sized human male—and without ever lifting weights. Cats, apes and many other animals instinctively stretch and flex their muscles using isometrics, pushing against both themselves and the outside world.

This being the case, the origins of what we call isometric exercise are surely lost in prehistory. Ancient Greek wrestlers used isometric principles in their training, for instance by squeezing and holding grips and locks for extended periods of time, and even pushing or pulling against pillars, walls, trees or each other. Isometric principles are visible in ancient martial arts such as Kung Fu, which utilize the body's muscular counter-tension, focusing on tightening the core of the body and becoming centered. The legs, in low stances, push down against the Earth and lift the torso upward from within, as the limbs extend outward with isometric power. In classical Yoga, muscles are actively flexed and contracted even as they are stretched and extended. A kind of natural traction—stretching, opening and extending the spine—is created by the isometric counter-tension of the body's muscles. In the past two hundred years, strongmen such as Eugene Sandow, Max Sick and Charles Atlas have popularized various systems of isometric exercise. Like the ancient Greeks, the Indian yogis and the Asian martial artist masters, they have tried to understand, express and convey the concept of muscle control—the idea that your mind-body connection can allow you to literally control your muscles at will and tap into your maximum physical potential. Modern Brazilian Jiu-Jitsu practitioners are able to control their muscles with great subtlety, allowing them to fight and defeat much larger opponents; we also see the incredible muscular control and development of bodybuilders, whose posing routines show off excellent control of isometric contraction. Watch a bodybuilder's posing routine sometime, and notice the way a top bodybuilder can completely isolate his leg, back or arm muscles. However, that's not the end of the game: ultimately, everyone who craves physical excellence will try to forge a deeper mind-body connection. Isometrics is both a great place to start and a path to real excellence; and as you develop awareness, feel and control of your muscles, you'll begin to see that the possibilities are limitless.

Antagonistic muscles and muscular efficiency

In a sense, many of the skeletal muscles are positioned to work *against* each other: one pulls one way, and the other pulls the opposite way. Functionally your body moves by contracting one muscle group while relaxing the opposing muscle group. For example, if you throw a punch your triceps tenses and flexes—straightening your arm outward; simultaneously, you biceps muscle relaxes, allowing the arm to straighten with no resistance. For any body movement it will be more efficient to relax an antagonistic muscle group while its opposite is performing work. If two antagonistic muscles or muscle groups are simultaneously tensed then they are literally working against each other, creating drag. This is one reason why people with large bulky muscles aren't necessarily the best at a particular sport: the speed, quickness, efficiency and endurance of a champion athlete are far more dependent on precise control over the muscles than on their sheer bulk and strength. Of course big strong muscles can be good, but they are even better if you know how to use them with maximum efficiency. A secret of muscle control is that if you can effectively relax antagonistic muscles while exerting muscular force, you will effectively have greater strength, speed and endurance. Less drag equals a more efficient use of energy. This is a simple abstraction of course; complex movements involve many muscle groups simultaneously and consist of many fine shades and combinations of muscular impulses and responses. In sports, it is rarely as binary as "biceps contracts—triceps relaxes." But in essence the simple idea is true, no matter how complex the action: the better your knowledge, understanding and technique is, the better and more efficiently you will use energy and force while minimizing drag. This is one reason why a golf, tennis or singing instructor will often start out by telling you "Just relax."

Muscular contraction

A muscular contraction is the tensing, flexing and shortening of a muscle, all the way down to the cellular level. When a muscle contracts, its fibers are pulling inward, tightening, shortening and condensing. Contraction is the opposite of muscular relaxation, which is a "letting go" or releasing of muscular tension— taking your foot off the gas pedal. When muscles are relaxed, they lengthen easily. *External* resistance comes into play when, for example, you pick up a barbell weight and try to bend your arm with it, "curling" it with your biceps muscle. Your biceps muscle contracts, but the barbell you're holding adds resistance against the contraction of the muscle and the bending action of your arm: this resistance from the added weight makes your biceps muscle work that much harder, and it has to contract more forcibly and exert more energy in order to bend the arm. In fact, if the weight is heavy enough, you simply won't be able to overcome the resistance and lift the weight.

Isotonic vs. Isometric contraction

If we consider the above example of trying to curl a barbell that is too heavy, we can see that even when you've contracted your biceps with maximum power the muscle is not necessarily at its shortest point, as it would be if the arm was fully bent. The fibers of the muscle may be contracting with maximum force, but the biceps is not shortened completely unless the arm is fully bent; it may even be completely extended while the muscular contraction is occurring. We make an important distinction here between muscular contraction, even maximum muscular contraction, and the overall length of the muscle or a limb's position along a range of motion. Yes, you *can* maximally contract your biceps when your arm is completely bent; but you can also contract the biceps with equal energy and intensity when the arm is straight. The contraction of a muscle and the shortening of a muscle are not exactly the same thing. The contracted muscle is tensed, activated, flexed, squeezed and exerts force; and without any resistance, the muscle *will* shorten and will pull on the skeleton, causing movement. When a muscular contraction significantly shortens the muscle and moves the body, this is called *isotonic* contraction. The opposite of an isotonic contraction is an *isometric* contraction. Lifting weights or doing other kinds of resistance training is somewhere between isotonic and isometric work—you will be moving the body through resistance, which is more isotonic, and at points of muscular fatigue or failure you'll stop or strain at a fixed point, which is more like isometric contraction.

An *isometric* muscular contraction is a contraction that does *not* shorten the muscle or move the body. Regardless of your starting position, if you contract a muscle without significantly shortening it or moving your body, then that is an *isometric* contraction. An isometric contraction can occur when the body is pushing against an unmovable resistance such as a wall—your muscles are contracting, but neither you nor the wall are going anywhere. If you were to push the wall over somehow, then you would be moving through the wall and at that point, you're no longer doing isometrics. If you press your palms against each other and squeeze, you are essentially doing this kind of pushing-against-the-wall contraction: the muscles of your two arms are deadlocked, pushing against each other. Since the resistance is equal to the push, and since *you* control the amount of force, in theory you should be able to contract your muscles with *maximum* exertion, just as if you were in a gym lifting heavy weights, without moving your body at all. You can also create an isometric contraction within your own body by contracting a muscle in place and working against the contraction with a counter-action of antagonistic muscles: for instance resisting the contraction of the biceps with a simultaneous contraction or stabilizing action of the triceps. We can use both external and internal resistance in our isometric work, and there are sophisticated tricks of body mechanics and leverage we can use to zone-in on and work specific muscle groups effectively.

Isometrics explained

The practice of isometrics can be defined as a form of exercise that is performed by contracting muscles or muscle groups without moving the body. The word "isometric" itself combines the prefix "iso" (same) with "metric" (distance), with the implication that in isometrics the length of the muscle doesn't change during the contraction, as contrasted with an isotonic contraction, in which the length of the muscle does shorten.

When you utilize the principle of isometrics for exercise, you are consciously flexing, contracting and *working* your muscles without moving your body; this requires, first of all, mental focus and body-awareness. In contrast to a sport or activity like tennis or jogging where you just "do" the activity, and the exercise is a kind of side effect, when you practice isometrics you are getting pure, intentional, targeted muscular contraction; you're working your muscles directly using isometric technique and the power of your own mind.

The key concept to understand about exercising and developing your muscles isometrically is that it is always the focus, intensity and quality of a muscular contraction that matters—not body movement, "maxes" or "reps." For example if a weightlifter lifts a big barbell into the air this may not necessarily in reality exercise his muscles very efficiently at all. He may be lifting the weight very *efficiently*—but our goal is not to lift weight, it is to work the muscles. If you have to move a bunch of heavy furniture, you should strive to be as efficient as possible. This is functional efficiency. However, if your goal is to work your muscles as much as possible, this requires a different kind of efficiency and a different kind of mindset:

now you want to generate the highest quality and the highest intensity in your muscular contractions. From this perspective if I can "max out" my muscles in 15 minutes or even less then that's *great*; I *want* the benefits of a workout and I want to get stronger and I want to feel good, so the sooner the better—my goal isn't to keep exercising all day and make it last. The difference between "functional efficiency" and *isometric efficiency* consists in placing the emphasis on getting the highest quality muscular contractions versus doing the most work. We can illustrate this by comparing somebody who curls a 30-pound weight 20 times, to somebody who curls a 10-pound weight only 3 times, but in a very slow, targeted, and focused manner, yet exerts his biceps muscles twice as much. The second lifter isn't trying to lift the weight quickly or efficiently, he is trying to generate powerful sustained contractions in his muscles, to really work those muscles out. He is lifting the weight very slowly and stopping along the way, holding the weight while flexing the biceps muscle isometrically with a lot of focus and intensity—he's using isometrics in his weightlifting workout, incorporating isometric contraction within a range of motion.

Again, the difference lies in placing the primary focus on working the *muscle*, not on the muscle doing work. Of course, there's some overlap here, and developing isometric strength will make you more efficient and stronger athletically; but from the perspective of isometrics the key element is the targeted and sustained intensity of the muscular contraction. Taking this idea a step further, we can now see how we could generate the best possible muscular contractions even up to the level of *maximal* muscular exertion without moving the body at all. By means of static resistance, muscular counter-tension, or both, it is possible to work your muscles effectively and to improve your strength, endurance, health, attractiveness, well-being, and even your mental focus and mood. You can work off *tons* of stress, adrenaline and aggression by pitting your own muscles against each other, and letting them in effect wrestle and fight each other, all of them getting stronger and *smarter* in the process. When you understand isometrics you can get *all* of the benefits of working out at the gym without going to the gym; you can easily get an intense *isometric* workout virtually anywhere and anytime, at your own pace and in tune with your own body—and get *real* results. Anybody, even those with serious disabilities or injuries, can vastly improve their overall muscle tone and muscle control. The possibilities are limitless. Again, think about the big jungle cats. They never lift weights, ever, but they have the most fantastic muscle tone, strength and agility that anyone can possibly imagine. Watch a cat stretching or flexing, and you will see a perfect demonstration of isometrics in action.

Muscle control and the Mind-Body Connection

Practicing isometrics, you will learn to consciously isolate and control your muscles, which strengthens the connection between your mind and your body. Ultimately, this *mind-body connection* is not something trivial; it's a rabbit hole that leads to deeper and deeper levels of self-awareness and self-control. Everyone controls their muscles with their mind already, to a greater or lesser extent, whether they are particularly aware of this process or not; when we seek to extend and enhance this conscious control of our bodies we find that we discover even more than what we had originally bargained for. Mental awareness of your muscles develops naturally as you practice—you'll start to really notice how your muscles *feel*; and in the same way you've learned to flex and contract your muscles, you also learn to relax them, and to *release* muscular tension. You will begin to find answers to questions like "Just how does my mind tell my muscles what to do?" The answers to these types of questions are ultimately beyond verbal description and the scope of this book, and exist instead in the domain of experience, intuition and personal feeling. However, one thing is certain: a deeper awareness of your body will open up new levels of your personal potential and your enjoyment of life. It's not an exaggeration to say that some of the concepts and techniques we will be studying in this book are derived from the most advanced and esoteric teachings of yoga and the martial arts. The possibilities are endless.

Types of isometric contraction

1. Isometrically contracting a muscle by pushing or pulling against something immovable; for example a tree or a wall.

2. Isometrically contracting a muscle by resisting with force from your own body; for example pressing your hands against each other as you flex your arm muscles.

3. Isometrically contracting a muscle while you apply counter-force internally with an antagonistic muscle; for example holding your arm straight with your triceps while you simultaneously contract your biceps isometrically.

4. Isometrically contracting a muscle as you stretch it; for example pressing your palm flat against a wall with your arm extended straight, as you simultaneously flex your biceps, or touching your toes as you isometrically contract your hamstring muscles.

5. Isometrically contracting a muscle from it shortest, fully contracted position; for example bending your elbow completely, and then flexing and squeezing the biceps.

6. Isometrically contracting a muscle as you extend outward, *lengthening*; for example flexing your quadriceps as you extend your leg out through your heel, or isometrically flexing your back muscles as you sit up straighter, lengthening your torso upward. Here you are isometrically flexing a muscle as the contraction works in synergy with related muscle groups to effect a lengthening action—you are contracting the muscle isometrically, but in such a way that the contraction has a *lengthwise pulling* effect.

Relaxation is a key

The opposite of muscular contraction is relaxation. Contraction is a kind of tensing; a tightening, an inward squeezing, a shortening—relaxation is the opposite. As you learn to forcefully contract various muscle groups in a targeted controlled way it's only natural that you will also develop the ability to relax those very same muscle groups. If you can learn to effectively *flex and tighten* a muscle at will, then you'll also become increasingly aware of whether a particular muscle is tensed or relaxed. As you practice isometrically contracting your muscles more and more, you'll be able to make increasingly subtle internal distinctions between muscles that are tight and contracted, or loose, supple, and relaxed.

Many people walk around in an unfocused state of constant muscular tension—this is a major component of stress, which is a major factor in many ailments including high blood pressure and insomnia. Stressful emotions and memories can "freeze" muscular tension in the body; and if a stress stimulus is severe enough or constantly repeated, this type of chronic tightness and tension can last years or even decades. Stress can literally etch itself into the fabric of your body over time, shaping *who you are* through the muscular tension you carry with you; at some point it becomes unclear if your body is tense because of your stressful emotions, or if you have stressful emotions because your body is so tense.

It's only natural that as you begin to master the concept of muscular tension and contraction in your own body, you'll also gain an awareness of its opposite, physical relaxation. As your awareness of muscular tension and relaxation expands, the implications for your entire being are profound. Isometric work can burn off stress and adrenaline and expend the excess energy stored in your muscles; this in itself is calming, and goes a long way toward helping you overcome Tilt and conceal your tells. However, learning to explicitly release and relax your muscles is just as vital; you will increasingly become aware that truly and completely relaxing your muscles can unleash incredible power.

Slow sustained muscular contraction

A secret of isometric training is that a mild or moderate muscular contraction held for an extended period can be very effective in strengthening and conditioning a muscle. An intense isometric contraction is not always what is required; a *light or moderate* isometric contraction can work very well also. The crucial factor, in this case, is that the contraction is *sustained*. A prolonged, moderate contraction can, in its own way, work a muscle just as effectively as a briefer, more intense contraction. Try flexing your forearm, but not too intensely: squeeze your fist gently, focus your awareness on your forearm muscles and lightly flexing them. Continue to breathe normally. Afterwards, deliberately relax your hand and forearm, even though you didn't really exert much force. Breathing regularly and staying relaxed during isometric work is one of the key components of proper technique—it helps you to avoid straining and it helps you to maintain normal blood pressure; it also allows you to sustain isometric contractions longer. If you lift weights you might be accustomed to a kind of "breathe in, push as you exhale" type of breath rhythm. That's NOT what we're doing here: we're getting away from pushing the muscles with the breath, and we're learning to control and flex the muscles *independently of the breathing action*. We generally start a contraction with an in-breath, then exhale smoothly while holding the contraction, and then continue to breathe normally as we hold the contraction longer, keeping the rest of the body relaxed. The intensity of the isometric contraction is something that we can adjust, upward or downward, as desired.

Fast twitch muscular contraction

Another weapon in your arsenal is the ability to rapidly flex and release a muscle repeatedly for a series of fast repetitions. An example would be rapidly clenching and unclenching your fist under the table; here you're using your rapid response or "fast twitch" muscle fibers to quickly switch on and switch off the muscular contraction. This develops a slightly different type of muscular control, and you might find that by employing this technique you can quickly get a "burn" or a "pump" in your muscles, especially if you squeeze fast *and* hard. You're also improving your ability to instantly accelerate from zero to full intensity, taking a muscle from its relaxed state to a full power contraction very rapidly and returning it a relaxed state just as rapidly. For most techniques, we will generally use a smooth and sustained isometric contraction; however, the rapid-fire flex can be a highly effective variation.

Poker Isometrics

What is Poker Isometrics?

There are many reasons why poker and isometrics go together well:

1. Sitting at a poker table is an excellent position from which to practice isometrics.

2. Isometric exercises don't require you to move your body, strain, breathe heavily or sweat.

3. Poker often requires players to sit patiently during a game for extended periods; burning off your excess energy with isometrics makes it easier, more enjoyable and healthier.

4. Playing poker well requires emotional control and a steady, level temperament; isometrics provides a powerful outlet for "Fight or Flight" stress responses and aggression, giving players a real handle for controlling stress and emotional reactions.

5. Because poker requires so much patience, a poker player has many opportunities to channel extra time and energy into practicing and mastering isometrics.

6. Physical poker tells are usually the result of involuntary physical responses; a player who is actively engaging his muscles with isometrics will give off fewer involuntary clues—and will tend to mask and conceal his emotions and feelings more effectively.

Isometrics can have substantial physical benefits, and sitting at a poker table is a near ideal scenario for sustained practice. On top of that, isometrics can actually improve a player's emotional control, patience and mental balance. As a poker player, if you can dramatically improve your strength, muscle tone and long term health, all without interfering with your schedule, and even improving your game while you're at it, then that is definitely +EV.

Poker Isometrics is stealth isometrics

 In poker, the ethos of deception and self-concealment runs deep. Being deceptive is an integral part of being a good player. Poker is a game of incomplete information and managing the information you give off at the table is crucial: opposing players are always trying to read your actions, your words and your overall affect to give themselves an edge in their decision making. Are you bluffing? Do you have a super-strong hand? Are you on a draw? In a live game, opposing players will be using every fiber of their being to try and figure out what your hand is, and they *will* be looking at your body—your hands, your face, your eyes, your neck, your shoulders, your legs—to try and get more information about what you have. The stereotype of the unreadable poker player who can successfully bluff in impossible situations is a big part of poker-lore and the poker image, and always will be.

Poker Isometrics is stealth isometrics; Poker Isometrics is covert and concealed. The whole concept of Poker Isometrics revolves around the fact that its practice is sneaky and unseen; it is always camouflaged, inconspicuous, unnoticed and disguised. If you practice Poker Isometrics correctly, *no one* will know it. As you study the techniques, keep in mind that there are always two goals:

1. Working the muscles effectively
2. Disguising and concealing what you are doing

All of the techniques of Poker Isometrics mimic or adapt common body positions you would reasonably see at any poker game; and the idea is to blend in the isometric muscle work seamlessly, so that nobody notices it. Because Poker Isometrics is secret and unnoticed, you have unlimited freedom to practice as much as you want without drawing any attention to what you are doing. Having acquired this skill, you can then practice Poker Isometrics essentially anywhere: waiting for a flight, riding on a subway, sitting in a meeting, doing a television interview, it doesn't matter. With good technique, it won't be noticeable to anybody that you are practicing isometrics, even if they're watching you rather closely. So you can always get in some work on your arms, pump up your calves, or burn off some stress if you feel like it.

Correct Poker Isometrics technique begins with breathing: continuing to breathe smoothly while holding an isometric contraction is fundamental Poker Isometrics technique. Continuing to breathe normally during an isometric technique allows you to target specific muscle groups while keeping the rest of your body relaxed. It will also moderate your blood pressure, and prevent you from straining. You may be flexing your biceps isometrically at *peak intensity*, but because you continue to breathe smoothly and evenly, the rest of your body won't tense up and your face won't strain or turn red. This allows you to work your muscles much more efficiently, and to hold your isometric contractions much longer; it also goes a long way toward concealing what you're doing. The techniques of Poker Isometrics have been designed with stealth and concealment in mind; as you learn to work your muscles effectively with the various techniques, keep in mind this central concept of stealth.

Poker Isometrics technique guidelines

Here are the fundamental technique guidelines for practicing Poker Isometrics. As we progress further into the book and begin presenting multiple variations and subtle adjustments, you should nevertheless always follow these guidelines. These guidelines are essential, not only for keeping a low profile when you do isometrics at the poker table; they're also essential to the effectiveness and to the safety of your practice.

1. **Breathe naturally.**

    As we've already mentioned, continuing to breathe smoothly and naturally will help you keep your body relaxed and to maintain normal blood pressure while contracting your muscles isometrically. This simply cannot be overstated: breathing naturally during isometrics will allow you to practice more effectively, with more focus, and to hold your muscular contractions longer and conceal what you're doing. Do NOT hold your breath when working your muscles with isometric contraction. Like a kettle letting off steam as the water inside heats up, breathing is a natural safety valve that allows you to work your muscles intensely without spiking your internal pressure.

2. **Keep your neck and face relaxed.**

    It is very important to remember when practicing Poker Isometrics to not tense up or strain your face and neck. Keep your face and your neck relaxed. There are several reasons for this—you don't want to drastically increase your blood pressure or the blood flow to your head, and you also don't want to look like you're sitting there straining at the table, like a constipated person sitting on the toilet. Also, we want to make a habit of *focusing* and controlling isometric tension in a specific muscle group while keeping the rest of the body relaxed. Maintaining a relaxed face and neck is a good place to start. Keeping your face and neck relaxed is also essential for concealing what you're doing.

3. **Target specific muscle groups in isolation.**

    In Poker Isometrics it's essential to isolate specific muscles or muscle groups. For example if you're working on your biceps, concentrate and focus the isometric contraction inside your biceps muscle. Try *not* to tense up the surrounding muscle groups, such as your back, triceps, shoulders and forearms. This is actually easier said than done, as there *is* a natural tendency when flexing a muscle for the surrounding muscle groups to get "recruited" into the contraction as well—muscular tension tends to spread into adjacent muscle groups. Also, some involvement of nearby muscles will often be necessary to stabilize a position or provide resistance and counter-tension.

However, as much as possible, strive to focus your isometric contractions into a specific muscle or muscle group; it's precisely at this point that your skills will improve as your muscle control develops. In some of the advanced techniques we'll be working with combinations, for instance working the upper shoulders and the back together, or the biceps and the chest, but the same principles will still apply: narrowing the focus of your isometric contractions to specific muscle groups will allow you to get the most targeted and most effective isometric workouts.

How to begin mastering isometrics using this book

As you read this book, take time to study the diagrams, illustrations and descriptions carefully. The visual images are designed to not only show the positions, but also the directions and interrelations of muscular force and counter-force. Often a subtle change in the angle or rotation of a body part makes all the difference for a technique. Think about what a specific technique is meant to do, and try to feel what your muscles are doing and how they react to various adjustments. Experiment, practice, and see what you can find.

1. Look carefully at the body positions in the photographs. Pay attention to subtle differences, such as the inward or outward rotation of a forearm. Attention to detail will fast-forward your progress significantly.

2. Think about how techniques target specific muscle groups. Look for similarities between techniques, as well as possible combinations. Read between the lines.

3. Carefully observe the directional arrows in the illustrations, which show points of isometric contraction and the direction of muscular force. The relative size of the arrows compared to each other generally indicates the relative intensity of muscular force. Clusters or pairs of arrows pointing directly at each other generally indicate isometric muscular contraction at that point.

4. All the isometric techniques are intended to be done while holding your body in a stationary position.

5. Be aware of the idea of muscular counter-tension. If one muscle is contracting, what other muscles are *countering* that contraction? Look for points of counter-tension in the positions, where your muscles engage each other and work against each other.

6. Listen to your body. Embrace the idea that isometrics involves a very real mind-body connection: *your* mind and *your* body. Ultimately, you will learn the most from feeling how your body responds, and what your body is telling you. Try to let your mind go *inside* your muscles, to feel, understand, and control what they're doing.

The simple isometric contraction

Here's how to do an isometric muscular contraction safely and effectively. You can always vary the intensity and the duration of an isometric contraction in various positions, but this is the basic, fundamental technique for isometric contraction in Poker Isometrics.

1. Focus your mind on the target muscle you'll be working on.

2. Inhale. Take a good deep breath.

3. Isometrically contract the target muscle, flexing and tightening it without moving your body. Hold your body steady as you squeeze and contract the muscle.

4. Keep holding the contraction, as you breathe out slowly, keeping your neck and face relaxed.

5. After exhale, either release the isometric contraction at that point, or keep holding it. If you do hold the contraction longer, allow yourself to breathe naturally. *DO NOT* hold your breath or strain your body.

6. When you let go of an isometric contraction, explicitly relax the target muscle. Breathe, and as you breathe, let go of the tension in the muscle. Try to breathe *into* the target muscle, with the idea of letting the muscle completely let go and relax.

As we progress in this book we will delve much further into the subtleties of isometrics, including advanced techniques, positions and adjustments that will skyrocket your progress and results. There is a lot to get to; but these basic steps are the framework for practicing all of the techniques that will be presented and described. Breathe in before you start. Focus on and isolate the muscle or muscle group to be worked on, and keep the rest of your body relaxed. Exhale and allow yourself to breathe during the isometric contraction. Release and relax the muscles afterword. This simple framework can be applied to all of the isometric techniques and variations in this book.

I am clarifying this point to eliminate any unneeded confusion or complexity. On the most basic level, this is how you do isometrics. There are no complicated sequences or mysterious breathing techniques or one-finger push-ups that you need to learn to *master* the techniques in this book. We follow this basic framework whether we are working on the arms, the legs, or any other muscle group. Likewise, whether we are doing very light isometrics or are contracting our muscles with maximum force, we still breathe naturally during the technique, focus and isolate the target muscles and consciously let go of the contraction and relax the muscles afterward. These same principles apply whether we contract a muscle for one second, or whether we lock a muscle into an isometric contraction and hold it for several minutes or even longer.

Again, our fundamental technique revolves around breathing naturally. Breathing naturally does NOT mean "Breathe in, flex, hold your breath, exhale." On the contrary, it means that you should continue to breathe naturally while you are flexing. Do not hold your breath during isometric contraction. Insisting on relaxed breathing during isometric technique, as well as working on isolated muscle groups separately and keeping the rest of the body relaxed, gives us the freedom to contract specific muscle groups very intensely if desired, and to hold those contractions for extended durations, without significantly elevating our blood pressure or straining our internal organs. By breathing, focusing and staying relaxed we can use isometrics very intensely, and at the same time safely, and covertly. This allows us to work specific muscle groups very effectively, at close to maximum exertion, and to get very powerful results, fast.

Visualization and body control

Visualization is a very effective way to enhance your isometric practice. *Visualizing* a technique in your imagination as you do it, requires you to become more aware of what exactly it is that you're doing, and thereby clarifies your understanding of it. Performing a technique *physically* doesn't mean as much if your mind isn't in it, so to speak; it's more valuable if you're mentally focused on what you're doing.

When you practice isometrics you are exploring and deepening your mind-body connection, and your mind gets stronger just as your body does. When you learn to isolate and flex a particular muscle, the part of your brain that controls that muscle is getting stronger, and you are etching new neural pathways into your nervous system. Your mental body image, a kind of virtual reality puppet in your mind, acquires more detail as your control over it strengthens. Imagine scratching your nose; now physically scratch your nose. Notice how in your mind's eye you performed the action before you *physically* performed the action with your body.

As you begin mastering isometrics, you will be learning to consciously control many of the muscles of your body and to flex and engage them in new ways. What you will be learning is how to control and work your muscles directly and explicitly: you *won't* be learning any sports, calisthenics, or other types of activities. You're learning to control your muscles in such a way that you can activate, flex and effectively work them while holding your body motionless. As you strive to master isometrics and to control your body, use visualization to your best advantage. This will in time become second nature to you and you won't really have to think about it. Visualize your muscles contracting isometrically as you flex them; visualize your muscles relaxing as you relax them; imagine letting go of your muscles and releasing all the tension in them. Sometimes, imagine that you are breathing *into* a muscle as you flex it, or as you relax it. Try to *see inside* your muscles—visualize the inner structure of your muscles, or an inner map, and try to line that map up with your body, always making that map better and more accurate. Your strength, muscle control and fitness will skyrocket.

The power of a single technique

 There are many isometric techniques in this book; but mastering isometrics is not a matter of memorizing hundreds of techniques. A teaching from Yoga is that a one good technique, if practiced, understood and ultimately mastered, can transform you. The idea is that every classical Yoga posture contains within it the key to mastering all of Yoga. In a similar way isometrics skill is deep as well as wide. You don't need to learn every technical variation in this book; you can begin getting good at isometrics almost immediately—learning and practicing even *one* of the techniques in this book correctly starts the process. You can get a lot of benefit starting out with one technique; a single technique, properly executed, can have tremendous benefits. If there's a technique that you find appealing or that's easy to remember or that you find enjoyable, then start off with that one, and try to do it correctly. A little bit of real isometrics goes a long way, and as you develop a taste for it you will naturally want more. My suggestion is that you allow yourself to learn from this book organically; as you progress, you'll begin to understand new concepts and how to use and combine various techniques for an even greater, more synergistic effect.

Safety rules for Poker Isometrics

1. Breathe normally when practicing isometric techniques, and do <u>not</u> hold your breath.
2. Keep your neck, face and head relaxed.

3. If at any point during a technique you experience a feeling of pressure in your head, or you feel dizzy, faint or lightheaded, STOP immediately. Breathe, relax, and consider getting up from the table and walking around for a few minutes.

4. Consult your doctor before attempting any of the exercises or techniques in this book, or before starting any new fitness program.

Benefits of Poker Isometrics

- Increased strength
- Muscle tone
- Muscle control and physical coordination
- Good posture and alignment
- Hormonal balance
- Relaxation
- Releasing stored muscular tension
- Natural outlet for the body's Fight or Flight response
- Tilt control
- Fighting boredom at the poker table
- Reducing impulsiveness and mistakes
- Concealing your emotions at the poker table
- Controlling and concealing involuntary poker tells
- Healthy blood pressure
- Good circulation and cardiac health
- Increased oxygenation
- Improved sexual response
- Better moods and increased mental focus
- Longer life and better long term health

There is an array of physical and mental benefits to practicing isometrics; and given the amount of time that many of us play poker, sit at a desk, drive or even fly, the opportunity is always there for us to add the benefits of *real* isometric practice to our lives. Poker Isometrics can seriously improve your game, also: you won't get as bored waiting for cards, you'll play fewer weak hands, you'll make better, less emotional decisions, you'll have improved focus during long sessions or tournaments, and you'll be steadier when you take a bad beat or start tilting.

Tilt control

In the poker sense of the word, Tilt refers to an emotional or mental state that affects your judgment and makes you play bad. When you're on Tilt you're not playing your best: your emotional and mental chemistry is altered, and this causes you to make bad decisions, strategy mistakes, loose calls, bad bets, bad folds and foolish risks. It's possible to get into a state of Tilt anytime that you're emotionally upset, but this effect is often amplified when you're sitting at a poker table in a casino and you have no choice but to suppress your emotions in order to maintain your composure and outward control. When you're driving, walking or working you can shake off a bad emotional state more easily. But holding yourself steady at the poker table can be more difficult. When you're sitting there surrounded by opposing players and you get frustrated, nervous, angry, depressed, anxious, or upset, it can create a kind of internal echo chamber of negative feeling. This can distance you from your usual sensibilities and good decision-making processes, and can lock you into a deepening, spiraling pool of unpleasant emotions and unclear thinking.

 Losing a big hand, taking a bad beat, getting unlucky, making a dumb mistake, getting teased or insulted or losing your temper in a poker game can temporarily wreck your composure and plunge you into a boiling kettle of emotional and mental agitation where you can, and will, make mistakes and play below your capabilities. It will often be very clear to your opponents when you're titled, and makes the effect even *worse*, as savvy opponents will challenge you, needle you, and play back at you more aggressively when they can see that you're tilting.

This doesn't end at the poker table, either: when you get emotionally upset and stop thinking clearly, and start making stupid mistakes, bad things can happen—whether you're trading stocks, drinking in a bar, driving in traffic, negotiating with a client, or breaking up with a girlfriend. When your emotions get out of control, your thinking becomes muddy, confused and unbalanced. This is where the worst mistakes can be made, and sometimes these mistakes are life-changers. For some guys, that can mean jail time, serious physical injuries, financial disaster, relationship meltdowns, getting fired, and more.

The first thing to understand about Tilt is that it's caused by your emotions, and your emotions originate in your body. Emotions are essentially the mental feelings you experience when your body goes through states of physical arousal such as happiness, anger, fear and surprise. If you find a big tarantula on your toilet seat in the middle of the night, you will probably jump back about 10 feet without even thinking about it; you'll feel a surge of adrenaline, a wave of shock, your heart will be pounding and you may even scream.

Before you've even *thought* about the tarantula verbally ("There's a tarantula on the toilet seat!") you are already having an emotional reaction. You didn't see the tarantula, think about it, decide you should be scared, and then jump back; on the contrary, your *body* saw the tarantula before you were even actually aware of it. This happens because your optic nerves have to pass through the more "primitive" sections of your brain, such as the Amygdala and the Hippocampus, before they ever reach the more complex image processing and thinking sections. Your emotions of fear and surprise are really just your mental state as your body reacts to the situation; like a rider on a terrified horse, you feel and experience your body's agitation, but it's *not* caused by your thoughts. Of course you can train your mind to react better to surprises and danger; and, conversely, it is also possible to scare or stress your body with your thoughts and imagination. But the point here is that your emotions are physical reactions occurring inside your body, and the quickest and most effective way to get a handle on them is by using your body.

In live poker games, competing for real money against determined opponents, it's very easy to become emotionally agitated and tilted. Making a mistake, taking a bad beat, getting unlucky, getting bluffed, getting tricked, insulted or outmaneuvered— there are many ways to get emotionally agitated at the poker table, and it's not always easy to dismiss it as merely a game. Sometimes it starts because you're tired, impatient and frustrated; other times it seems like you were already ready to go on Tilt as soon as you sat down, somebody just had to flip the switch for you. Whatever the situation, though, if you start feeling bad or letting your emotions overpower you, you won't be playing your best and you'll be in real danger of going on Tilt. Emotions are physical reactions, but when you're playing poker you often have to just sit there and endure it. The advantage of Poker Isometrics is that it gives you real tools to burn off extra adrenaline and stress, come back to your body, and keep your head in the game.

Isometrics combined with correct breathing can calm, oxygenate and energize your entire body, and can give you a solid handle to keep yourself together when things get stressful. Anger, frustration, anxiety, aggression and other stress responses are typically part of the "Fight or Flight" response spectrum, and the adrenaline, cortisol, norepinephrine and other hormones that flood your bloodstream at these moments are intended to prepare your body for *action*—now. Using isometrics gives you a *real* outlet for this unavoidable and inevitable surge of energy and physical readiness. When you flex your muscles isometrically, working them at times with maximum force and intensity, you are *instantly* releasing the physical impulses and energies inside you that beg to be released. In the long run, you won't suffer from the same chronic stress that afflicts most sedentary people, and you won't have to contort your mind trying to talk yourself down from stress, as you stew inside a cauldron of stress hormones.

Staying off Tilt is largely a function of managing your body's stress responses, and keeping your head in the game. In this sense, Poker Isometrics may seem like a kind of magic wand that can untangle the gridlock of stress responses and inactivity that can force you into Tilt. Additionally, because practicing isometrics teaches you to relax your muscles you'll become even better at keeping your cool, and less vulnerable to emotional disruption. Understanding your emotions and developing *real* emotional control is no trivial task, but learning how to let off steam with isometrics is a very good tool that can help a lot—it both increases body awareness *and* provides a wide-open outlet for your extra energy and will power. When your emotions can't torture you, you'll stay off Tilt more easily: you'll think more clearly and you'll play the way you know you can play.

Concealing your tells

Physical poker tells are generally involuntary, and you're usually not aware of them for the most part. They betray you without you ever even knowing about it. At other times you'll be aware of a potential tell—feeling nervous or scared when bluffing for example—and you'll try to cover it up by acting in the opposite way, in this case trying to act confident, relaxed, happy, aggressive or intimidating. The problem is that if your opponent is aware that you're trying to act or to "reverse your tells", that in itself will be a tell: a savvy opponent will be able to infer a lot of information if he perceives that you want him to see you in a certain way. In this sense, covering up or reversing your tells can be even worse than the tells themselves; like a suspected criminal who gets caught by the police returning to the scene of a crime to hide evidence, your attempt at concealment convicts you. The classic example, from Caro's Book of Poker Tells, is the "strong means weak" equation: a player with a strong hand will often act weak in order to lull his opponent, while a player with a weak hand will often act tough and aggressive to intimidate *his* opponent. Of course, if both you and your opponent are aware of the "strong means weak" paradigm and if you are both aware that the other knows about it as well, then the meaning of acting aggressively or meekly in a particular poker situation can change considerably. You might be acting aggressively thinking that your opponent will interpret it as a deception, or, thinking he could be aware of that possibility as well, you might be intentionally reversing the tell yet again, and so on. This starts to get into multiple level thinking and game theory—but the simple fact is that very well known and obvious tells, such as blustery aggression or demure meekness, cannot always be taken at face value because poker players tend to be tricky. In a live game you're generally better off trying to pick up subtle clues from your opponent's overall affect, and matching that up with other situational clues and information, such as betting lines. Sometimes your intuition will put the pieces together and you'll get a solid read. At other times the picture will be murkier, and it's best to base your actions solely on poker strategy.

This gets us back to the poker tells that you're not aware you give off. Blind spots can always be dangerous, and our unconscious physical poker tells are quite literally blind spots in our physical self-awareness. A perceptive opponent might be able to, for example, pick up on the fact that your neck tightens up and you lean your head to the right when you're bluffing, or that you slouch down in your chair when you bet and your hand can't stand a raise. Since you're not aware of these subtle, personal, idiosyncratic tells, it's difficult to suppress them. You generally can't see how you look to other people.

Poker Isometrics can give you a big advantage in concealing your unconscious tells. If you practice an isometric technique at the poker table you'll be more actively controlling your body, and you will, in a sense, override some of the random, undirected body movements or static which might otherwise be leaking information to your opponents. For example, let's say your tell is to tense up your neck and lean your head to the right when you're bluffing. If instead, at that moment in the game you're working your biceps isometrically, the undirected and habitual action of leaning your head to the right is less likely to occur, because you'll be actively working on your biceps muscle. Because you're *actively engaging* your body, you'll give off fewer unconscious tells, and the "tells" that your opponents might *think* they perceive will tend to be incidental, and therefore meaningless to what is occurring in the game. Additionally, since the practice of Poker Isometrics burns off stress and enhances your ability to control and relax your body, you'll just generally be better able to maintain your composure and conceal your tells in tight spots. Actively using Poker Isometrics will tend to replace and override habitual tells and fidgeting that may happen when you're trying to sit still under pressure; and because your muscle control and relaxation skills are improved, your overall body control game will be improved as well.

Poker Isometric Biceps

The biceps is located on the front of your upper arm and extends between the shoulder and the elbow. It's the powerful muscle that bends your elbow, and you use it when you pick something up or pull something toward you. The biceps muscle is paired antagonistically with the triceps muscle: the biceps flexes the elbow and *bends* the arm, and the triceps extends the elbow and *straightens* the arm. The biceps and the triceps pull in opposite directions and naturally resist each other—this why coaches tell boxers to relax their arms when punching to increase speed: if the arm muscles are relaxed there's less resistance and drag created by the opposing muscles, and so the punch travels much faster.

When using isometrics to work the biceps, we need resistance; sometimes we employ the counter-force of the triceps to hold the arm steady, and sometimes we use our opposite hand to resist. However, in both cases, we are contracting the biceps muscle isometrically, working the muscle without changing the position of the arm or the bend of the elbow. This is isometrics: we contract the biceps muscle but we do not shorten the muscle or move the body. The ability to hold your arm stationary while isolating and contracting the biceps muscle isometrically with control and focus, will allow you to get an intense biceps workout virtually anywhere and anytime.

When we work the biceps while holding and resisting with the opposite arm, the biceps is pulling upward against the downward pressure of the other hand, and we can exert maximum force up against this resistance. Think of flexing the muscle *first*; the muscular contraction generates the pull against the resistance, and not the other way around. This idea is crucial when we lift weights or use resistance machines at the gym: we flex the muscle (contraction), and it is flexing the muscle that lifts the weight—we let the pure muscular contraction lift the weight. Our goal is always intense muscular contraction and working the muscles, *not* lifting weights. Obviously in pure isometric practice there are no weights to lift at all... just muscles to contract, but you get the point.

When we work the biceps with *internal* resistance, the muscle will contract differently depending on the angle of the elbow. If the arm is straight, the biceps will be stretched tighter as you flex it; if the arm is completely bent, the biceps can be fully contracted— squeezed inward from its shortest position; and if the arm is partially bent the isometric contraction will vary along with the angle of the elbow and the counter-tension of the triceps. Experiment with different arm angles, as well as different durations and intensities. You'll find subtle differences between positions, such as the tendency of the biceps to cramp up slightly sometimes when maximally contracted, or the involvement of the elbow tendons and forearm muscles when contracting the biceps with a fully extended or stretched arm. Various subtle tweaks in the technique can have powerful effects on your results, so don't just gloss over them. Mentally connect with your biceps muscles using isometric technique and you'll be able to get pumped up anytime you want.

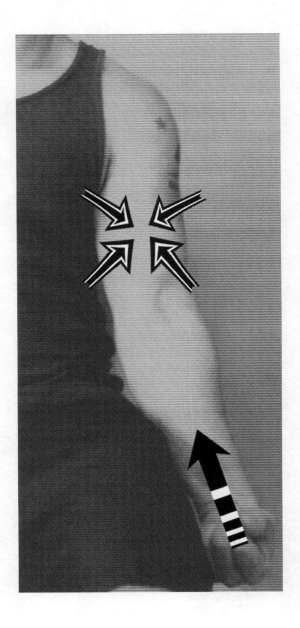

Hold your arm straight and flex your biceps muscle, as if you were curling a heavy weight upward.

Follow the basic *isometric technique guidelines*:

1. Breathe in as you contract the muscle.

2. Focus the contraction in the biceps.

3. Hold the contraction as you exhale.

4. Breathe naturally while you continue to hold the contraction.

5. Release the contraction, breathe, and consciously allow the biceps muscle to relax.

Feel free to experiment with varying intensity, duration and number of repetitions. Remember that quality counts for more than quantity.

Isometric contraction of the biceps with no external resistance: Bending your wrist up toward you, flex your biceps isometrically. Adjust the contraction by straightening your arm—squeezing the biceps as you pit the extension of your elbow against the biceps contraction.

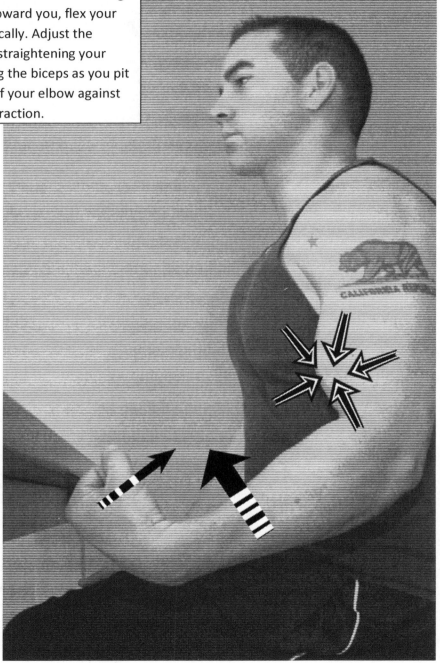

Isometric contraction of the biceps *with* external resistance: In this technique, you push down with your top hand and flex your biceps isometrically as you work to bend your lower arm upward against the resistance.

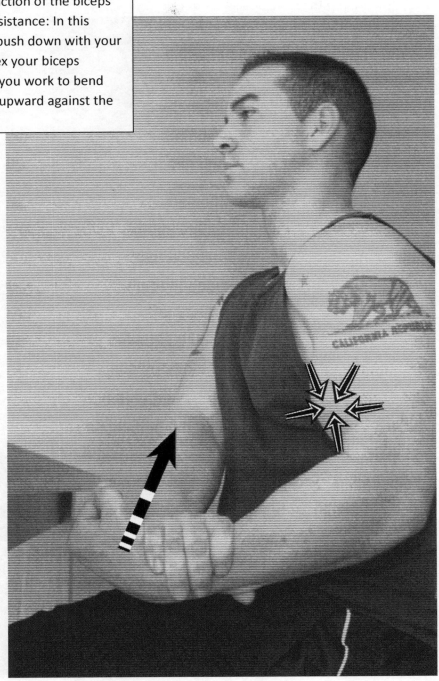

As a variation, try leaning your body into the table or backward away from the table, while pulling upward with your biceps against the resistance of your other hand.

Experiment with using a *mild*, *light* isometric contraction of the biceps, as well as a more intense contraction. Breathe.

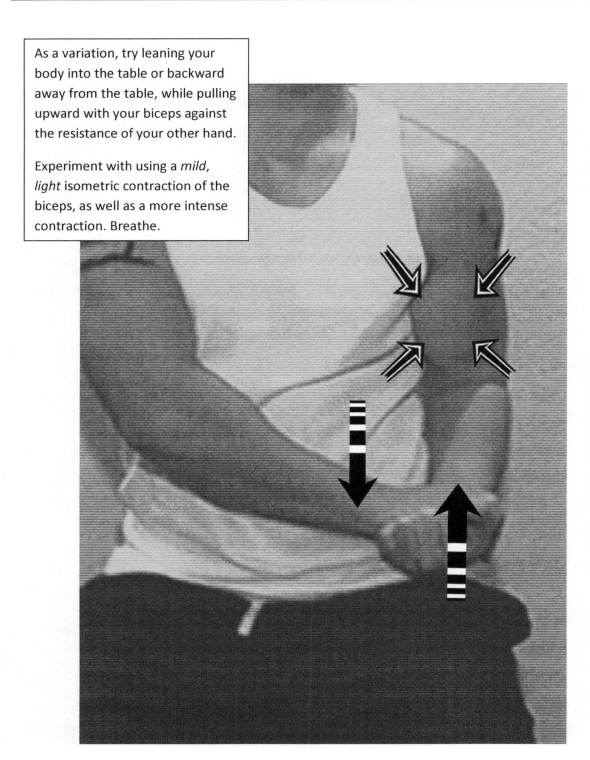

Now, position your hands in front of you; pull straight upward toward your chest, flexing your biceps isometrically as you resist, pressing downward, with your other hand. *Squeeze* the bicep. Breathe.

Now pull your hands across to the far side of your body and lean back as you pull your bottom hand upward against your top hand, flexing your biceps muscle, as your arms wrestle against each other; focus on the isometric contraction in your biceps. Turn your bottom wrist outward, to add some *twist* and to intensify the flex as you hold this position.

Now hold your elbow off to the side, creating a space between your ribs and your arm. Your top hand now presses outward at an angle against the bottom wrist. Hold the contraction in the biceps muscle as you allow your arm to straighten slightly. This will create a pulling action on the biceps. Notice that if you sit up *straighter* while keeping your hand in the same position you'll feel an added *stretching* action in your biceps as you flex it.

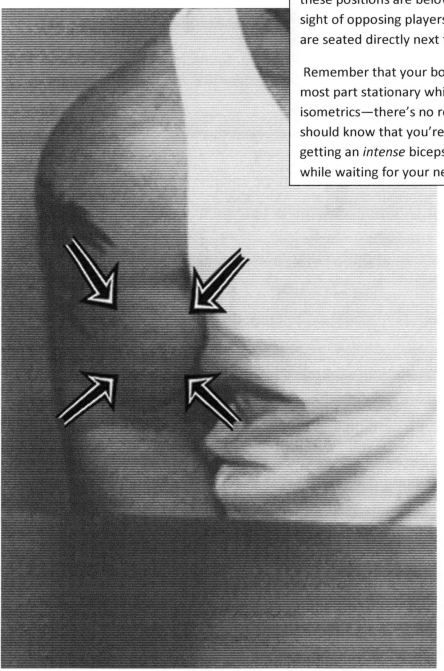

Notice that at the poker table, all these positions are below the line of sight of opposing players unless they are seated directly next to you.

Remember that your body is for the most part stationary while isometrics—there's no reason anyone should know that you're actually getting an *intense* biceps workout while waiting for your next hand.

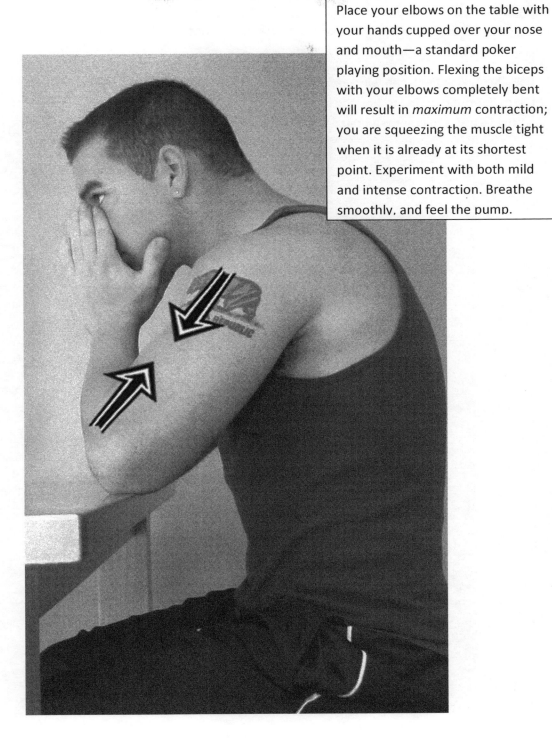

Place your elbows on the table with your hands cupped over your nose and mouth—a standard poker playing position. Flexing the biceps with your elbows completely bent will result in *maximum* contraction; you are squeezing the muscle tight when it is already at its shortest point. Experiment with both mild and intense contraction. Breathe smoothly, and feel the pump.

Now place your hand on the side or the back of your head, as if you were brushing your hair back or massaging your neck.

Again, flexing the bicep with your arm fully bent is a *powerful* contraction; ease into it, remembering to breathe naturally, and don't overstrain. If your biceps muscle starts to cramp-up, release the contraction and straighten your arm.

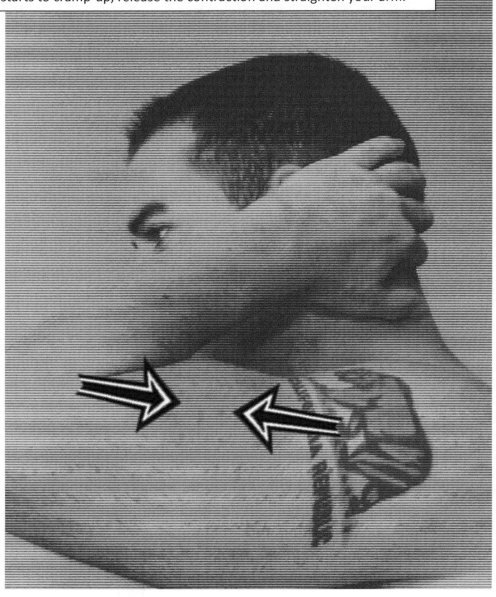

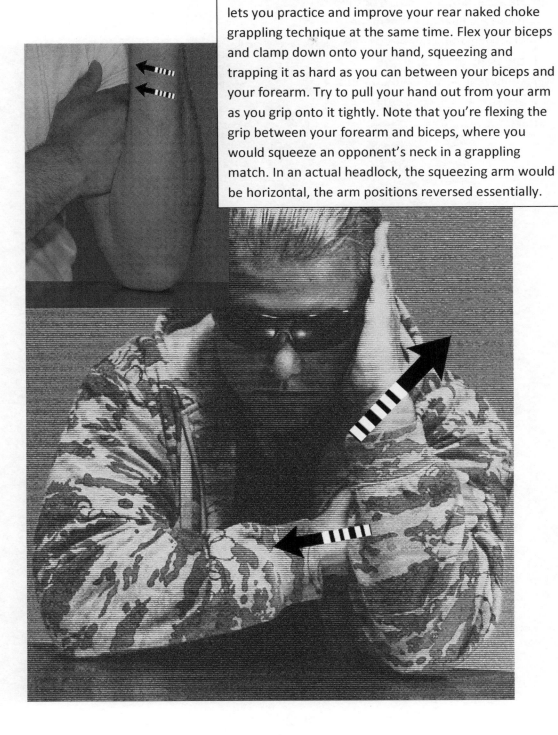

This is the isometric headlock. It works the biceps and lets you practice and improve your rear naked choke grappling technique at the same time. Flex your biceps and clamp down onto your hand, squeezing and trapping it as hard as you can between your biceps and your forearm. Try to pull your hand out from your arm as you grip onto it tightly. Note that you're flexing the grip between your forearm and biceps, where you would squeeze an opponent's neck in a grappling match. In an actual headlock, the squeezing arm would be horizontal, the arm positions reversed essentially.

Here's another variation of the isometric headlock technique. This time grab your biceps with the trapped hand, as you squeeze it between your biceps and forearm, flexing your biceps isometrically.

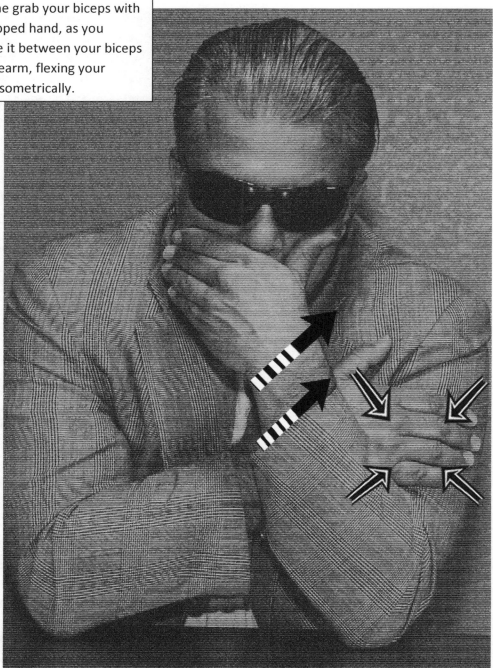

Here you're pulling on your elbow with your opposite hand, as you squeeze your biceps muscle isometrically, bending your arm as tightly as you can. Lean forward to increase the intensity of the contraction.

Reach one hand behind you, twisting slightly away from your arm with the elbow on the table. Flex your biceps isometrically, bending your arm as tight as you can.

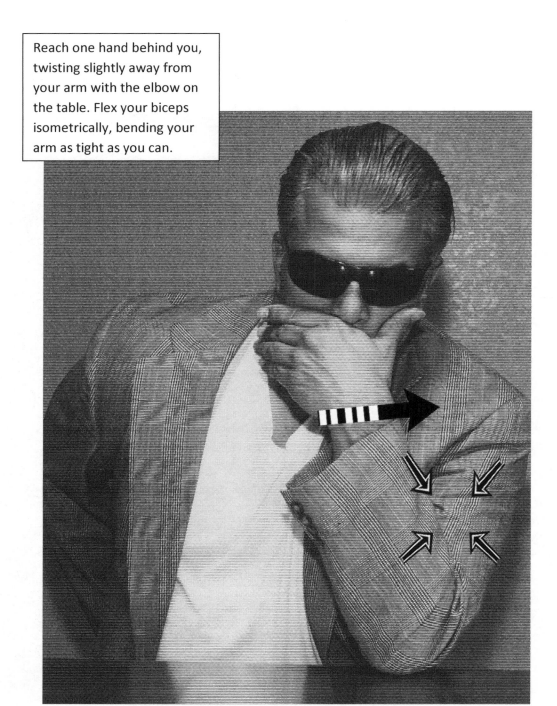

Grab under the table with your hand, and pull upward against the underside of the table. Flex your biceps as you lift *lightly* against the weight of the table with your fingertips and squeeze the biceps. You're *not* trying to lift the table here, you're just bracing yourself against it for resistance as you isolate and flex your biceps isometrically.

Breathe normally, focus on your biceps, and keep the rest of your body relaxed.

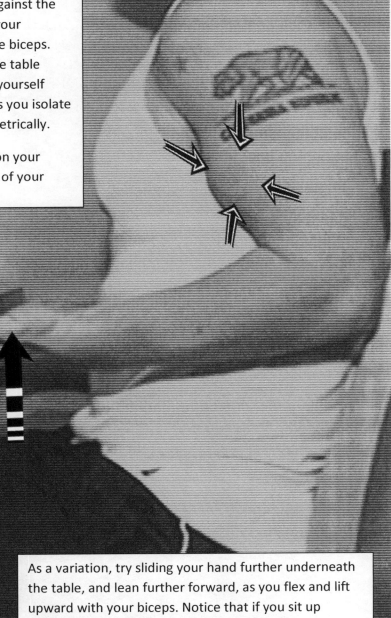

As a variation, try sliding your hand further underneath the table, and lean further forward, as you flex and lift upward with your biceps. Notice that if you sit up straighter from your waist at this point, you will automatically exert more pull against the biceps.

Now, bend your wrists *backward* as you flex your biceps; notice how the wrists bending backward adds resistance against the biceps as they pull upward. This is a somewhat *twisty* isometric technique that can burn a lot of extra tension and adrenaline *quickly*. Work fiercely against yourself to generate intense isometric contraction.

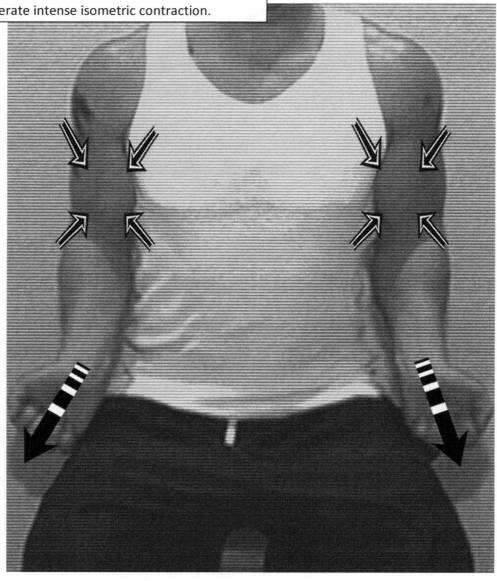

Isometric Chest

The muscles of the chest feel great when they've gotten a good workout, a good *pump*. The natural endorphins and the increased blood flow in your chest muscles after some intense isometric contractions can be positively intoxicating. Practicing Poker Isometrics you'll find that you can get an incredible chest workout easily while sitting in your favorite game. When you use isometrics to work your chest muscles think about <u>squeezing</u> the muscles inward toward your sternum to increase the contraction; notice the interplay of your arm and shoulder position as you flex your chest. You need to concentrate to isolate and effectively flex your chest muscles without moving your body around; *anybody* can work their chest doing pushups or bench-presses, but it takes *real* muscle control and body-awareness to get a major league pump while sitting at a poker table, in an apparently relaxed posture.

As you start practicing these techniques, focus first on the positions that work the easiest for you. If you find that when you try a particular technique you really feel it strongly in your chest muscles right away, then focus on that technique for a while and really master it. As you practice more and more, you'll start to develop a better feel for how the chest muscles work; you'll begin to find things that you didn't notice before, and at this point the subtle variations between techniques will become clearer, and you'll find new possibilities opening up for you. Experiment with low, medium and high intensity contractions, and experiment with short and long durations as well. Remember to *breathe naturally*; don't hold your breath, tense up your entire body or over-exert yourself. Focus on improving your ability to flex the chest muscles in isolation while keeping the rest of your body relaxed.

Notice how a slight adjustment to a technique, such as bringing your elbows closer together, can immediately intensify the effect of a muscular contraction. Pay special attention to the way the chest muscles can be squeezed and flexed more intensely when your shoulders move toward one another; observe the relation of your shoulder position to your chest muscles. Study the photos, diagrams and descriptions closely—subtle variations of angle, direction, pressure, posture and arm position can make a tremendous difference; and by understanding the distinctions between them, you will master isometric technique.

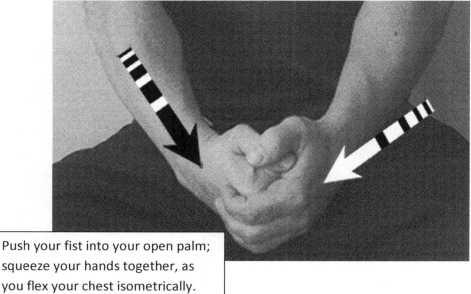

Push your fist into your open palm; squeeze your hands together, as you flex your chest isometrically.

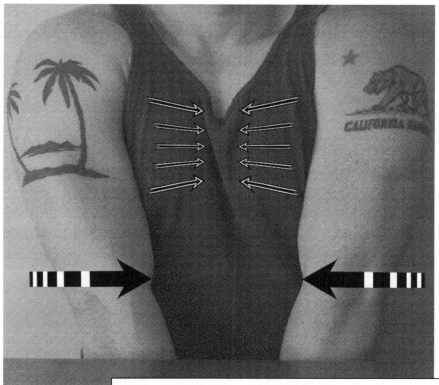

Pull your elbows closer together to increase the isometric tension, squeezing the chest muscles together.

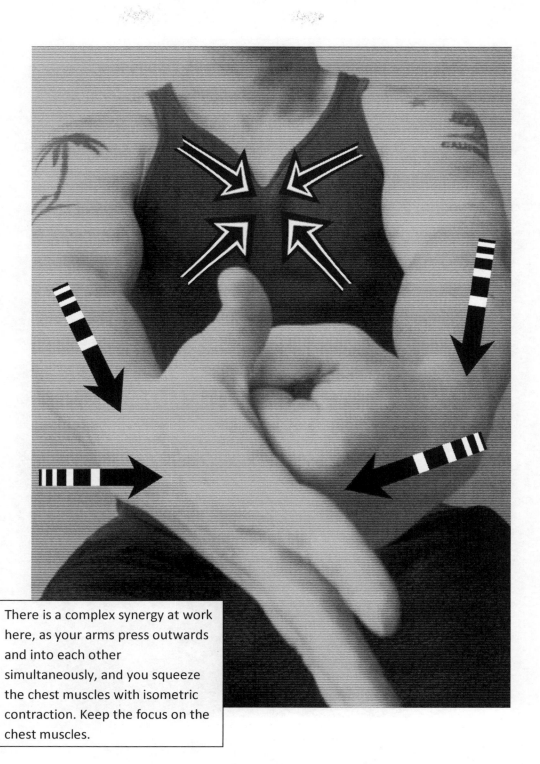

There is a complex synergy at work here, as your arms press outwards and into each other simultaneously, and you squeeze the chest muscles with isometric contraction. Keep the focus on the chest muscles.

Now squeeze your palms together using a Fireman's Grip and flex your chest. You can modify the contraction of the chest muscles by pulling your elbows slightly inward, closer to your ribs; or lifting them slightly outward, away from your ribs. Your two arms wrestle against each other—with the squeeze *starting* from your chest muscles.

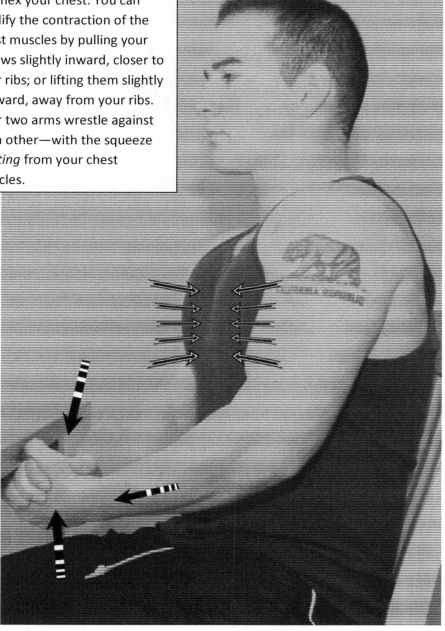

Now, still pressing the palms together in a Fireman's Grip, straighten your arms, bringing your elbows closer together. You'll notice *immediately* that this intensifies the flex of your chest muscles. You can adjust this position further by leaning slightly forward or backward, or by straightening your spine upward and lifting your head higher as you flex. Breathe.

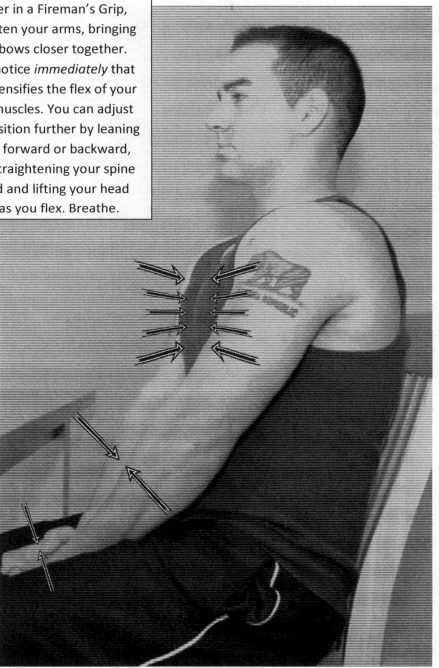

Now press your fingertips against each other under the table, while rotating your upper arms *outward* and pulling your elbows toward one another, as you flex your chest.

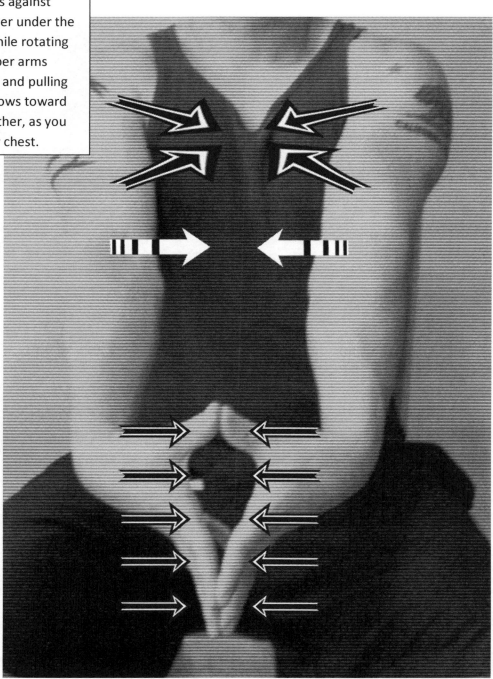

Now rotate your upper arms completely *inward*, so that the backs of your wrists are touching.

Squeeze your chest muscles with isometric contraction, as you push downward and press the backs of your wrists together, your hands curling away from each other.

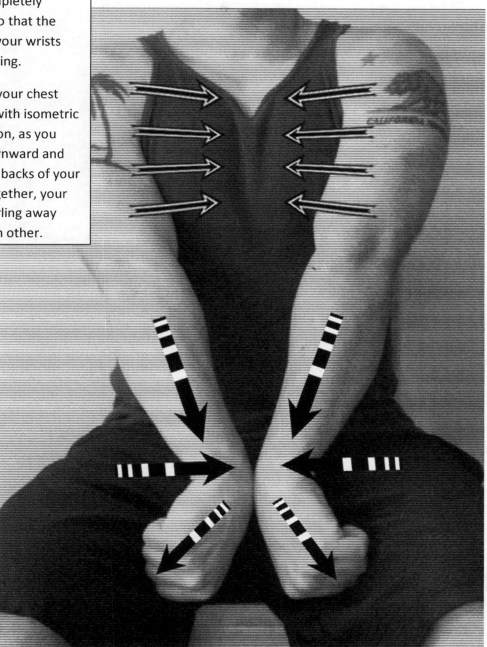

Press your palms together with your fingers pointed downward. Squeeze your palms together and flex your chest muscles. Intensify the contraction of your chest muscles by pushing your elbows forward while continuing to press your hands together. To add even *more* intensity, pull the inside of your wrists up toward your navel, while keeping your fingers pointed downward. Work within the power and synergy of the diamond shape formed by your arms. Focus the isometric contraction in your chest muscles, and allow the flex of your chest to push the hands against each other.

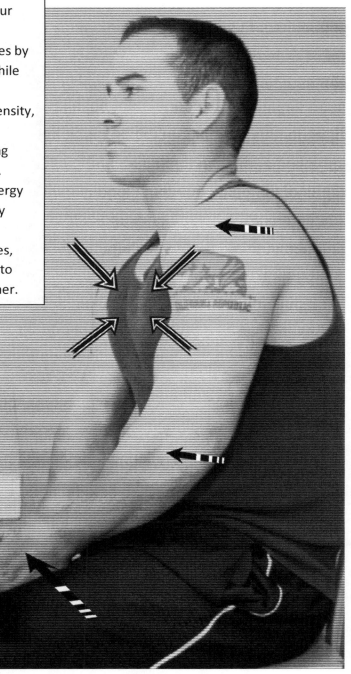

Now press your palms together with your fingers pointing upward. This can be done underneath the table with your hands in your lap, or discretely with your arms on the table.

Press your hands together as you flex your chest muscles with isometric counter-tension. You can adjust this position by pulling your elbows inward, closer to your ribs, or pushing your hands farther out in front of you; both of these adjustments will intensify the isometric contraction.

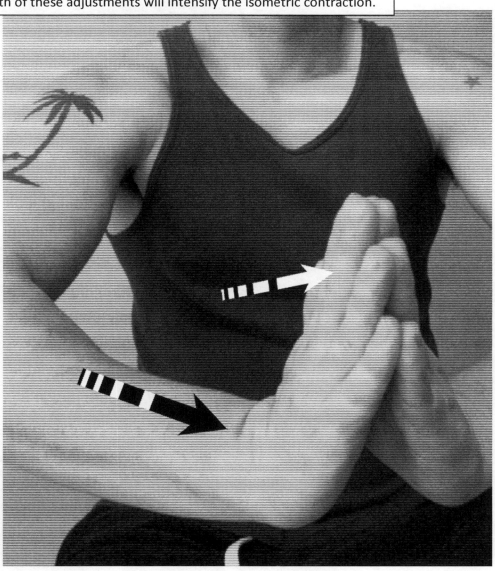

Press your fists downward between your legs, rotate your upper arms *inward,* and push your shoulders *forward* as you flex your chest. Squeeze your chest muscles together towards your sternum. Sit up straighter to increase the tension.

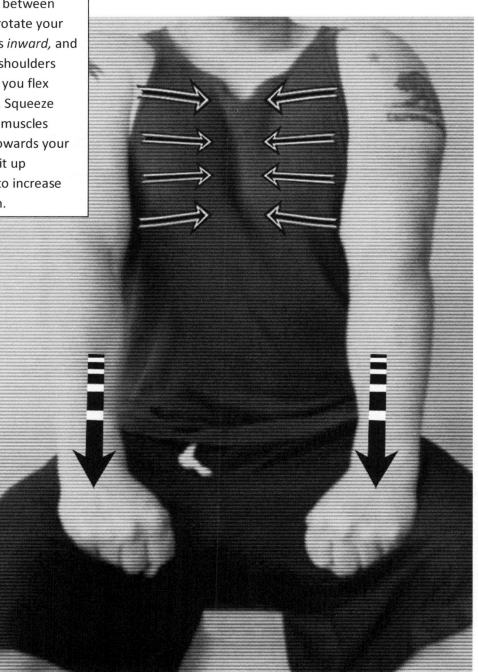

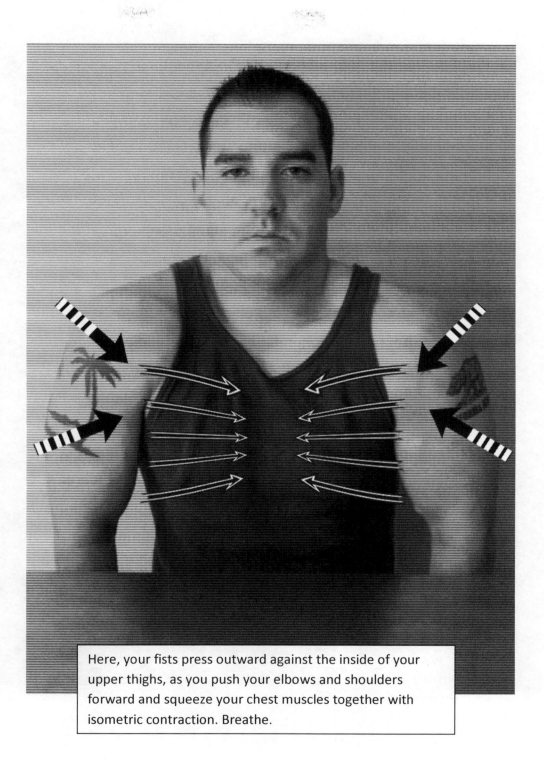

Here, your fists press outward against the inside of your upper thighs, as you push your elbows and shoulders forward and squeeze your chest muscles together with isometric contraction. Breathe.

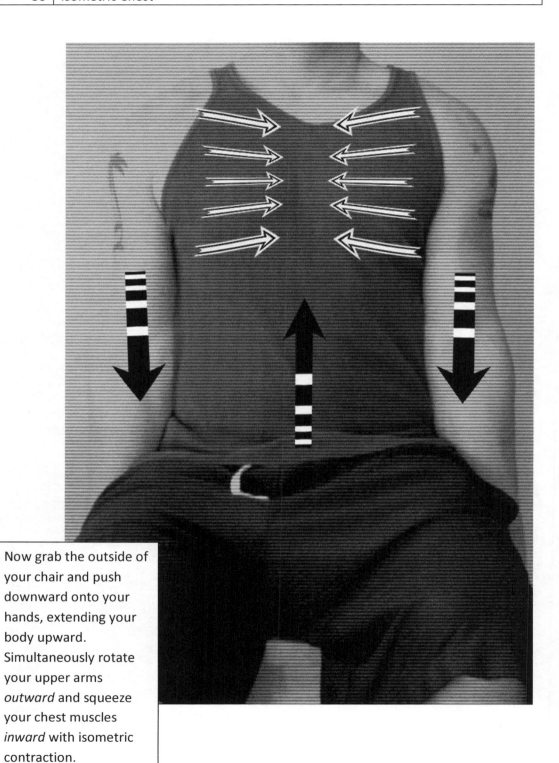

Now grab the outside of your chair and push downward onto your hands, extending your body upward. Simultaneously rotate your upper arms *outward* and squeeze your chest muscles *inward* with isometric contraction.

Press your fingertips into the outside of your thighs and push your shoulders forward, as you simultaneously squeeze your elbows in toward your ribs. Flex your chest isometrically, looking for the *sweet spot* of balanced counter-tension between the forward push of your shoulders and the inward pull of your elbows.

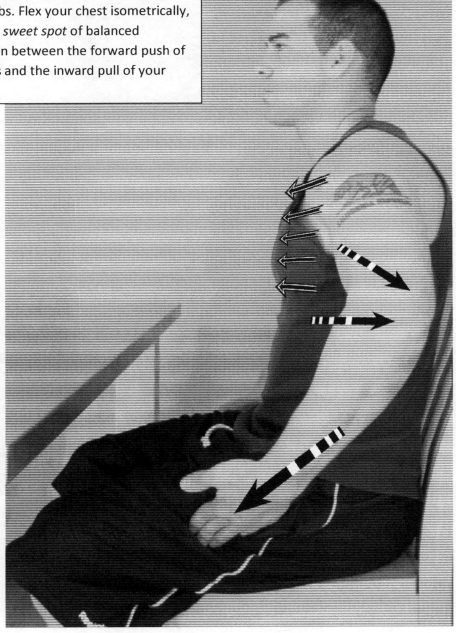

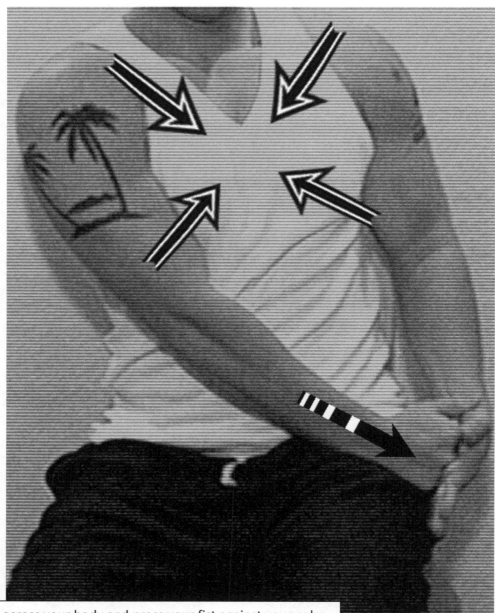

Reach across your body and press your fist against your palm, next to your far hip, as you flex your chest. You'll notice that this position engages your chest muscles very intensely. Isometrically *squeeze* the chest muscles.

For even greater isometric intensity, extend and straighten your arms off your hip as you press your fist into your palm.

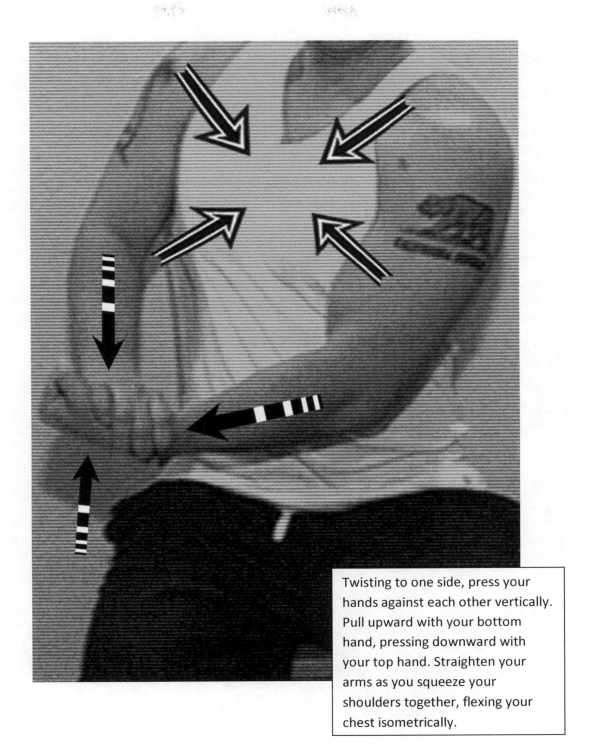

Twisting to one side, press your hands against each other vertically. Pull upward with your bottom hand, pressing downward with your top hand. Straighten your arms as you squeeze your shoulders together, flexing your chest isometrically.

Place your arm across your body and press your palm onto the table. Note that we are placing the *palm* on the table, *not* the elbow. This is a crucial distinction.

Flex your chest muscles isometrically as you twist your body *into* the crossed arm; you'll feel this working as soon as you try it. For even greater isometric tension, cross your *other* hand under the table and place it onto your *opposite* thigh. If you lean back from the table without moving your hands, the effect is even more intense. Breathe.

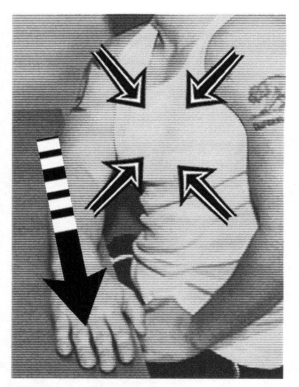

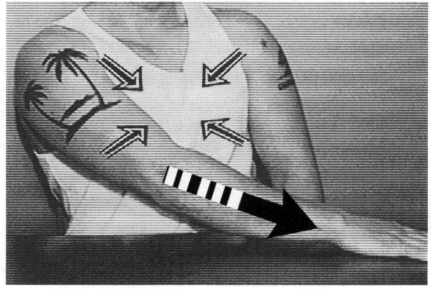

Place your hand on your opposite shoulder. Push your elbow across your body as you flex your chest muscles. Pull your elbow inward, closer to your chest, to intensify the isometric contraction.

Now grab your elbow and pull across your body as you flex your chest isometrically. Turn toward the *pulling* arm to generate more isometric tension. For best results, straighten the grabbed arm downward and brace it against your leg or the chair.

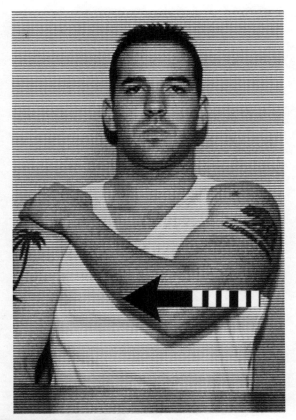

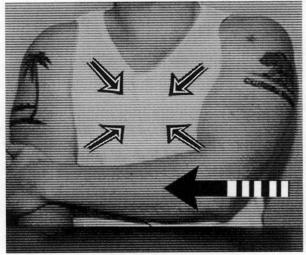

Here you're leaning forward onto the table, as if protecting your cards, and resting your head against your hand. Note the position of your elbows: the action here is to squeeze the elbows together as you engage your chest muscles with isometric contraction.

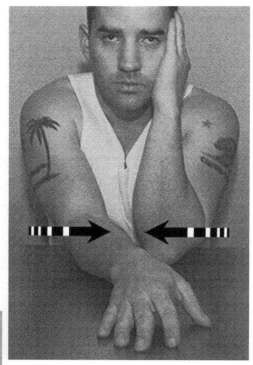

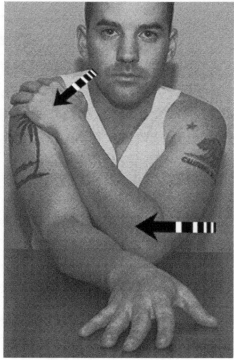

Here's another card protector variation: this time your hand is on your shoulder. Your elbows are again squeezing together, and the focus is again on flexing your chest. Lean back slightly without removing your hands from the table, and you'll intensify the isometric contraction.

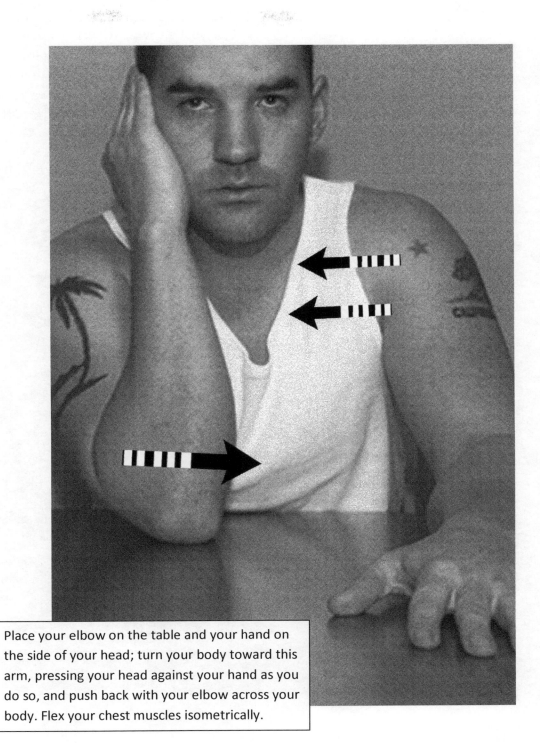

Place your elbow on the table and your hand on the side of your head; turn your body toward this arm, pressing your head against your hand as you do so, and push back with your elbow across your body. Flex your chest muscles isometrically.

Push your elbow across your chest with your arms crossed. Both of your shoulders push inward as you squeeze your chest muscles isometrically. The hand on the table presses downward, stabilizing the position and increasing the flex of the chest.

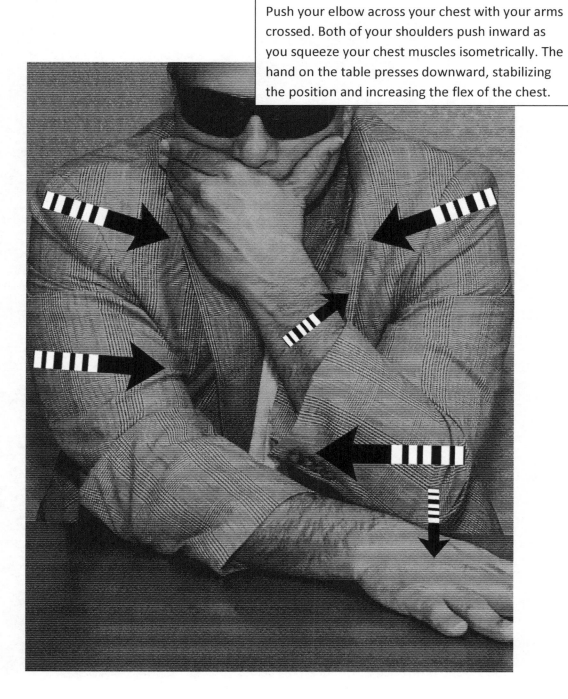

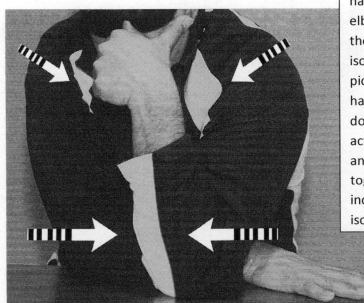

The top picture shows the elbow crossed in front of the hand; the shoulders and elbows squeeze together as the chest muscles contract isometrically. The bottom picture shows one of the hands extended pressing down onto the table; the action here is also the elbows and shoulders squeezing together. Sit up straighter to increase the intensity of the isometric contraction.

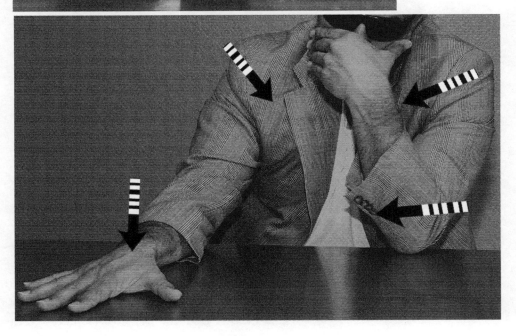

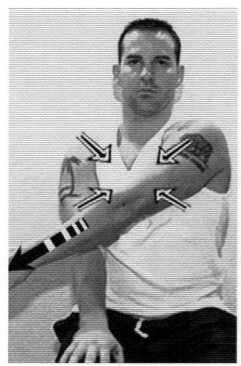

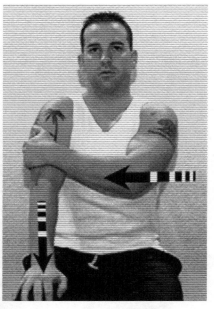

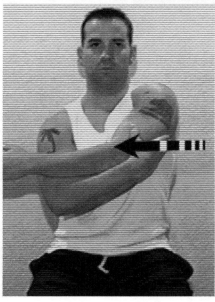

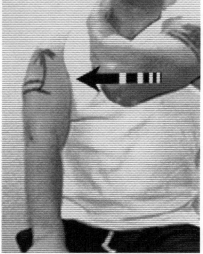

Here are a few more variations to experiment with. Again, look for the sweet spots of muscular counter-tension that generate powerful isometric torque.

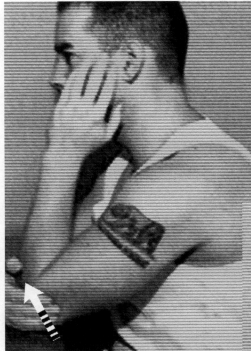

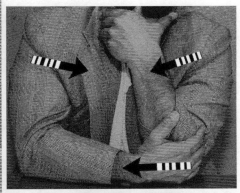

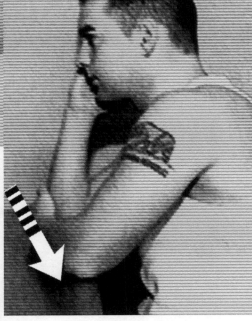

Here are a couple more variations that work the chest muscles with your elbow on the table. Pulling on your elbow with your opposite hand and squeezing your elbows, shoulders and pecs inward toward the center as you flex can be very effective—you have a lot of leverage against yourself, and you can intensely work the chest muscles from a stationary position. Turn *toward* the arm that you are grabbing, and place your elbow toward your center for best effect. These are all very common poker-playing positions that are *great* for isometrics.

Notice that you can create a sort of closed-circuit of muscle energy here—pulling on one elbow while pushing the other elbow outward: work within this isometric ring of power. Note the effect that sitting up straighter or leaning forward has on your flex.

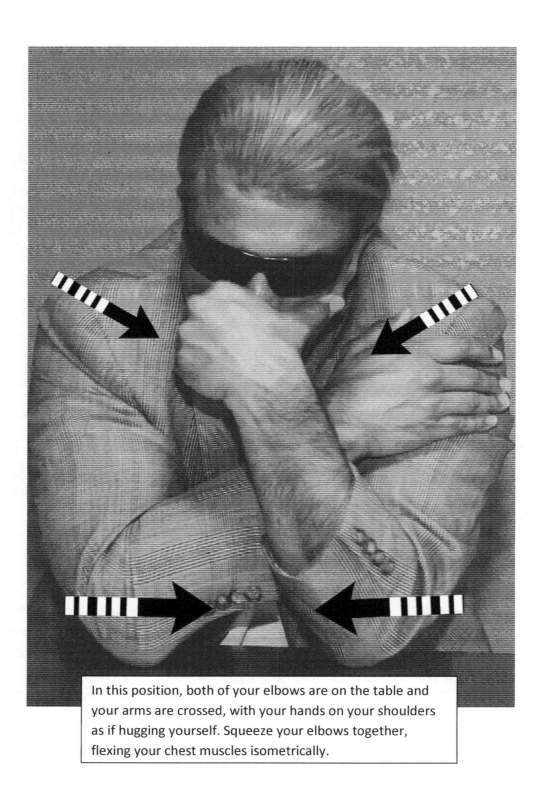

In this position, both of your elbows are on the table and your arms are crossed, with your hands on your shoulders as if hugging yourself. Squeeze your elbows together, flexing your chest muscles isometrically.

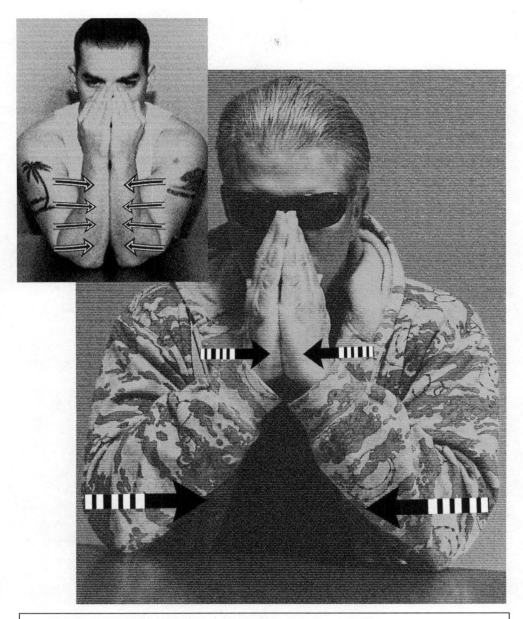

From a standard poker face-concealment position, squeeze your chest muscles, flexing them isometrically. Leaning back or sitting up straighter, without removing your elbows from the table, adds isometric tension. Placing the elbows together squeezes the chest muscles strongly when you flex.

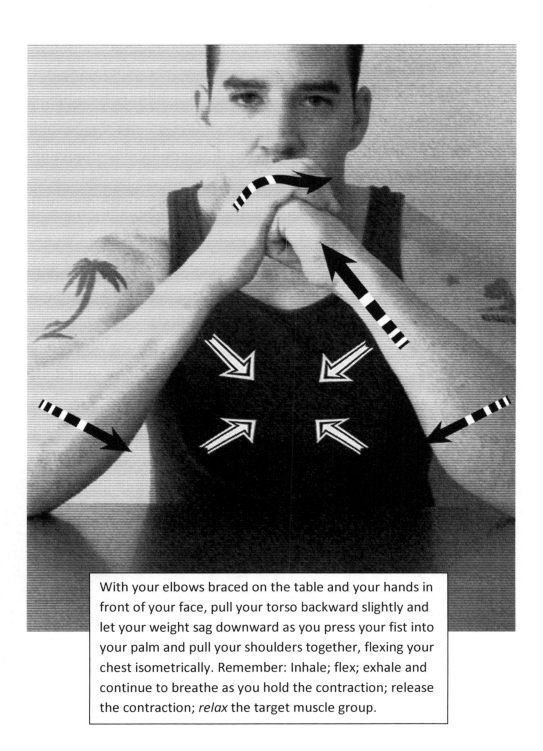

With your elbows braced on the table and your hands in front of your face, pull your torso backward slightly and let your weight sag downward as you press your fist into your palm and pull your shoulders together, flexing your chest isometrically. Remember: Inhale; flex; exhale and continue to breathe as you hold the contraction; release the contraction; *relax* the target muscle group.

Isometric Triceps

The triceps muscle is located on the back of the upper arm and extends from the shoulder to the elbow. When it contracts it extends the elbow and straightens the arm. The triceps muscle directly opposes the biceps, which bends the elbow joint.

When working the triceps using isometrics, sometimes we'll apply resistance with the opposite hand and work against it, and sometimes we'll flex the muscle in place with no external resistance, with the elbow either extended or partially extended. With the elbow completely extended and the arm straight, you can contract the triceps muscle fully, squeezing it inward on the back of your arm to its minimum length.

You'll find that isolating and flexing the triceps is a bit more difficult at first than working with the biceps. It might seem somewhat counterintuitive that as the triceps shortens and contracts on the *back* of the arm this action *straightens* the arm. Using isometrics the challenge is to flex these muscles on the back of the arm with the same intensity we generated with the biceps; when your arm is completely straight, it takes effort to engage the triceps isometrically—really flexing the triceps muscle and not merely continuing to straighten the arm. Working the triceps with the arm completely straight, you can intensify the isometric contraction by allowing the triceps to pull the arm slightly *shorter*, the triceps muscle lifting the back of the elbow up toward the shoulder. Try to find "grip" or traction with the triceps muscle on the back of your arm, so that you can sharply flex it and squeeze it isometrically, even when the arm is already completely straight.

You can also effectively *lengthen* the arm while flexing the triceps with the arm completely extended. With the triceps fully contracted and the arm straight, push out through the hand, lengthening the arm and *opening* the elbow joint. Be sure that you are not hyper-extending the elbow joint, but rather that you are in a sense stretching the arm lengthwise as you flex the triceps muscle, as if the muscles of the upper and lower arm were pulling the elbow apart and opening it. Play with the resistance and counter-force of this action, the simultaneous stretch and contraction of the triceps muscle and the engagement and strengthening of the elbow joint. If you practice this correctly, you can develop arm and elbow strength even at full extension, the point at which most people's arms are weakest.

Straighten your elbow as you flex your triceps muscle isometrically, as you press downward, *lengthening* the arm.

As the triceps contracts it *pulls* tighter on the back of the arm extending the elbow; lengthen your arm downward as a counter-action. Without leaning over, stretch your arm downward as if trying to touch the floor, as you sharply and firmly contract the triceps.

As a further adjustment, rotate your wrist and upper arm either inward or outward as you flex the triceps.

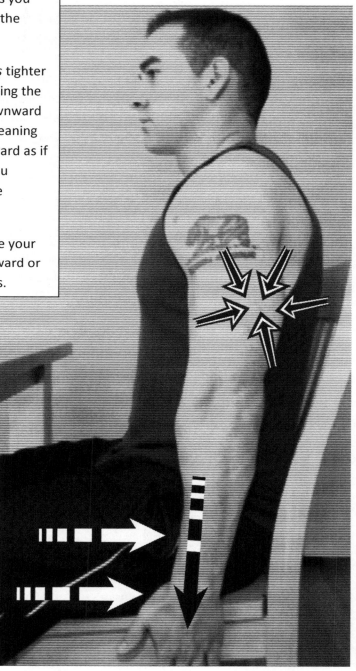

Now, as you extend your arm and flex your triceps, curl your wrist toward you. This adds yet another muscular counter-tension, as the elbow is extending, the wrist is pulling upward, the arm is lengthening and the triceps muscle is contracting isometrically *up* the back of the arm.

Think about increasing the strength of your elbow *at full extension*. This is usually the point in the arm's range of motion where the elbow is weakest and most vulnerable. We want to develop strength and control even with the arm completely straight—*feel* the pull between the upper and lower arm muscles, the balance of both the flexor and the extensor muscles, and the strength within the elbow joint itself.

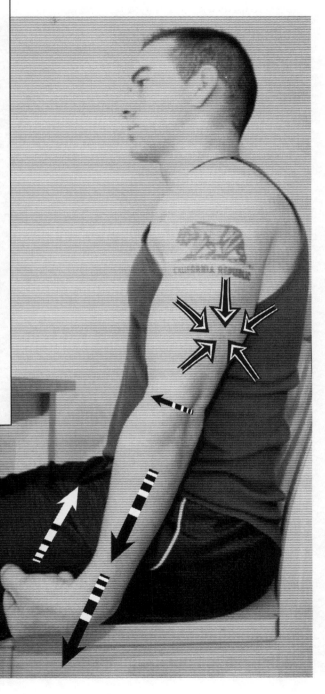

Here your lower arm is rotated so that your palm now faces *backward*. Curl the wrist towards the forearm, while extending your arm and flexing your triceps. As an additional adjustment, bend your arm very slightly to add more counter-tension to the triceps contraction. Keep the focus on the triceps muscle and the back of the upper arm.

Now twist your arm *outward*, as you extend it and push it backward, flexing your triceps *intensely*. Your wrist bends upward and your hand rotates *away* from your body as the arm extends; we're engaging the triceps here with an isometric *twisting* action.

Now your arm is extended completely behind you. Work to lengthen the arm further as you contract the triceps. Really *connect* with the isometric action of the triceps here—feel it tightening and pulling between your shoulder and your elbow along the back of your arm.

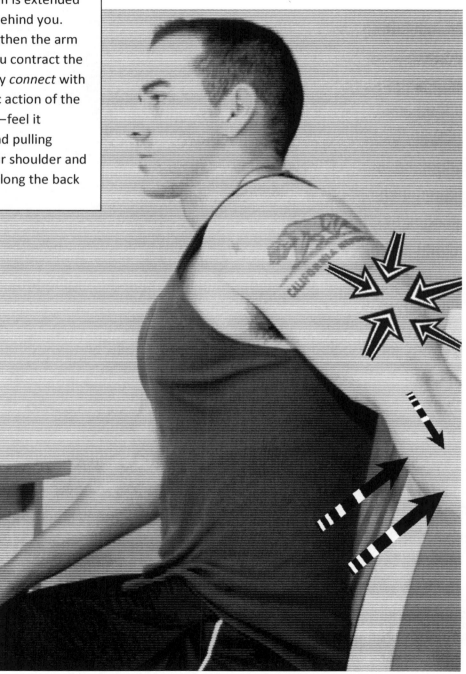

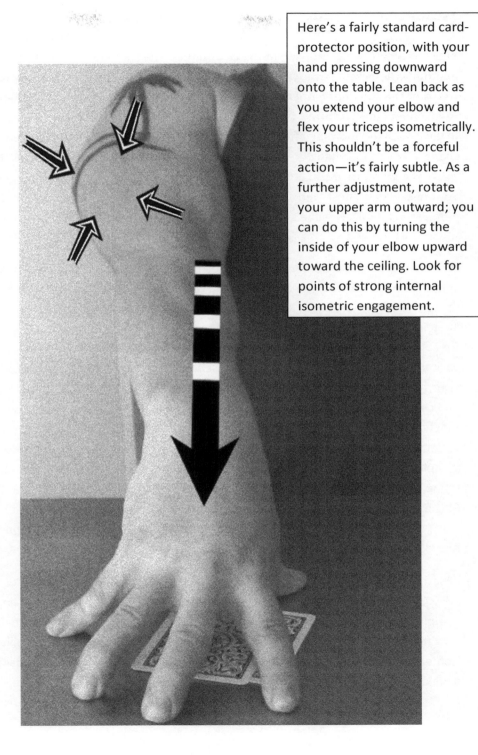

Here's a fairly standard card-protector position, with your hand pressing downward onto the table. Lean back as you extend your elbow and flex your triceps isometrically. This shouldn't be a forceful action—it's fairly subtle. As a further adjustment, rotate your upper arm outward; you can do this by turning the inside of your elbow upward toward the ceiling. Look for points of strong internal isometric engagement.

Isometric Shoulders

Your shoulders are comprised of the collarbones, the shoulder blades, the shoulder joints, and the various ligaments, tendons and surrounding muscles. Conceptually we could think in terms of the shoulder *girdle* extending from one side of the body to the other above the rib cage, connecting the arms, upper back, chest and neck. If you've ever woken up with a crick in your neck the morning after sleeping on a strange bed, you might've eventually found that the key to unlocking the neck pain had more to do with your *shoulders* than with your neck. The strength and alignment of your shoulders powerfully affects the well-being of your neck, back, chest, and spine, as well as your posture, body language and sex appeal. Females instinctively value strong shoulders, as they are powerfully masculine action muscles of the body.

When we work the shoulders using isometrics we involve many different muscles simultaneously; however in describing the techniques we'll often just refer to the deltoid muscle, the front or rear of the shoulder, the trapezius, or the shoulder blade area. Just keep in mind that we're describing the techniques in terms of functionality, and that when, for instance, we describe an isometric contraction of the shoulder or the deltoid, there are various inner shoulder muscles that are all interacting and flexing isometrically and working together in various ways. The descriptions of the techniques are designed to be as simple and clear as possible, so complex terminology is avoided, and the emphasis is on functionality. Study the illustrations as well as the descriptions—the adjustments and variations of the positions are designed to strongly engage the shoulder muscles. The complex interplay of the shoulder muscles can move the arms in every possible direction: lifting, pushing, swinging and rotating the arms every which way. This incredible complexity of the shoulders also allows us to use isometrics to great effect, flexing the shoulders in place and generating isometric counter-force from our arms, back, chest and the internal muscles of the shoulders themselves.

Experiment with the different techniques and variations; pay attention to subtle adjustments of angle and direction, and see how they affect your results. The shoulders are complex, and understanding them takes some effort. Many people never really think about how their shoulders work or what they do; what we're looking for is the ability to use isometrics to engage the shoulders powerfully from a seated, stationary position. Try to develop a feel for how to activate, flex and open your shoulders.

Lift your arm upward while resisting with downward pressure from your opposite hand. Lift *from your shoulder*, squeezing and flexing the deltoid muscle. Pull your *elbow inward*, closer to your side, as you flex your shoulder isometrically, intensifying the contraction.

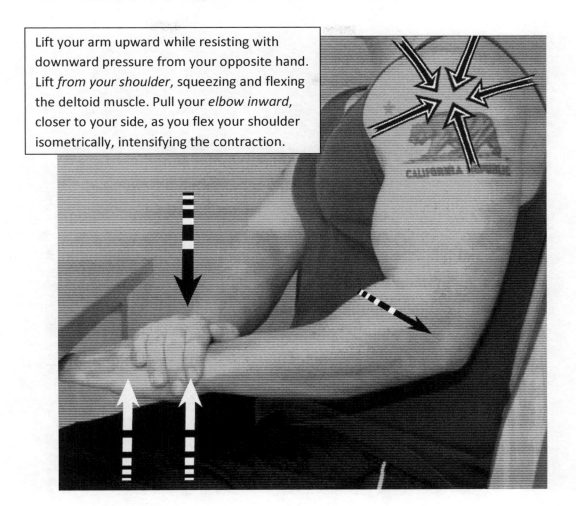

Remember that you are primarily flexing the muscle, in this case the shoulder muscle: this is not an exercise of pushing against your hand as hard as you can of generating a ton of force between your hands. Ideally, you want to target the contraction mentally, with the power of your concentration, in your shoulder muscle specifically. Placing your opposite hand over your wrist just gives you an extra point of kinesthetic engagement—in a sense it helps you "find" where that muscle is: the slight push against the opposite hand helps you locate the point of contraction in the shoulder and the angle of resistance helps you locate the muscular counter-tension. Of course, you can just apply pressure upward with one arm while resisting with the other; but keep in mind that the point is to actively flex and contract the deltoid muscle.

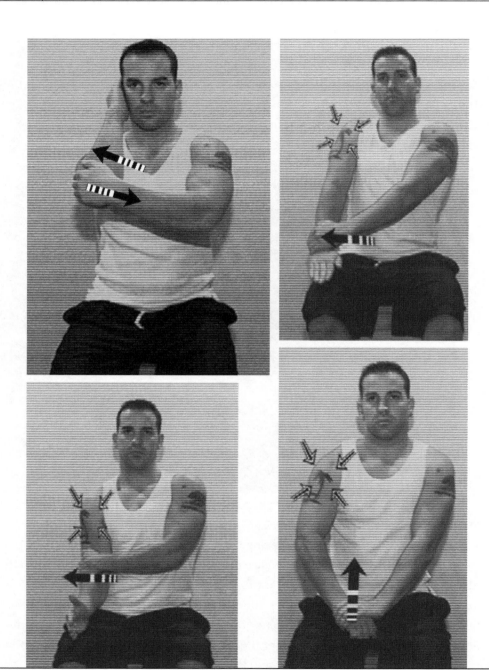

Here are some isometric shoulder variations—they all revolve around the outward or upward lifting action of the shoulder against the resistance of the opposite hand. These are all *stationary* positions and the focus is always on the contraction of the shoulder muscles.

Reach across your body and grab
the elbow of your opposite arm.
Flexing your shoulder, lift your
arm out sideways, while holding it
down with equal counter-tension;
this action engages the shoulder
muscles, especially the deltoid.

As a variation, rotate your upper arm
inward, so that the inside of your elbow
faces your ribs. Hold the back of your elbow
with your opposite hand and resist as you
lift your arm out *sideways*, flexing the
shoulder muscles with isometric tension.

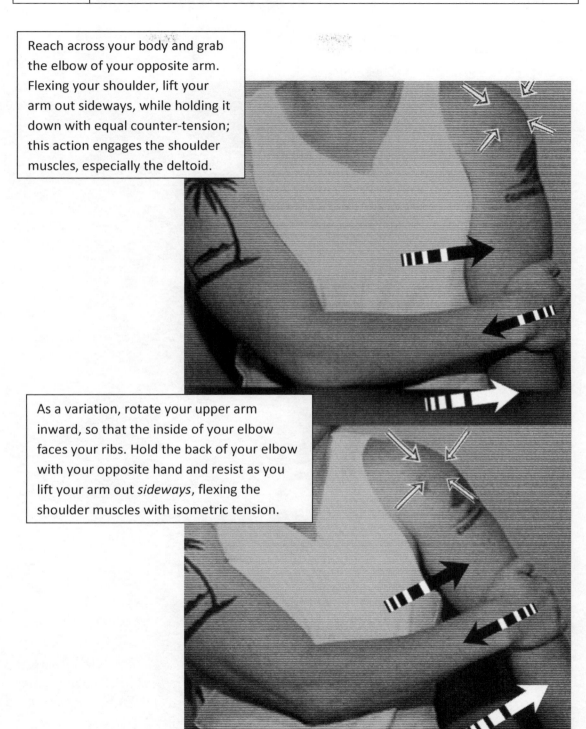

Press downward at an angle with your elbow, while resisting with your other hand and flexing your shoulder muscles isometrically. As a variation, you can interpolate and blend this downward action with an outward or upward isometric lifting action of your shoulder as well.

Here's another variation: with your hand at your head, pull your elbow backward and down, and resist by pulling against your arm with your opposite hand.

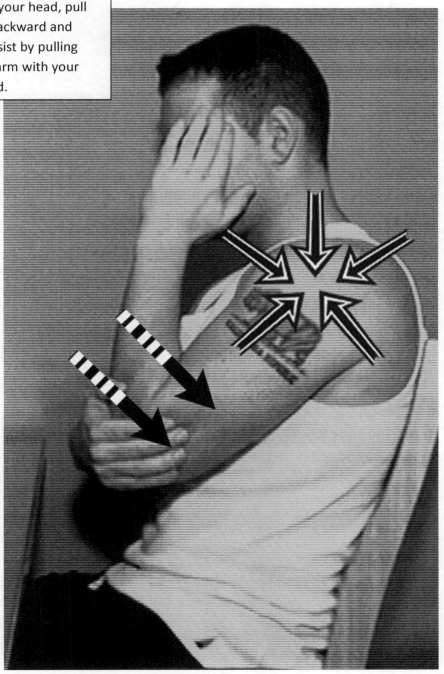

Place your palm flat on the table in front of you with your arm bent and your elbow pointing off to the side. As you flex your shoulder muscles, push the *outer edge* of your elbow upward, against the resistance of your other hand. The action of the shoulder is a lifting of the elbow *away* from the body and toward the ceiling; resist with the off hand and focus the isometric contraction in the shoulder muscles.

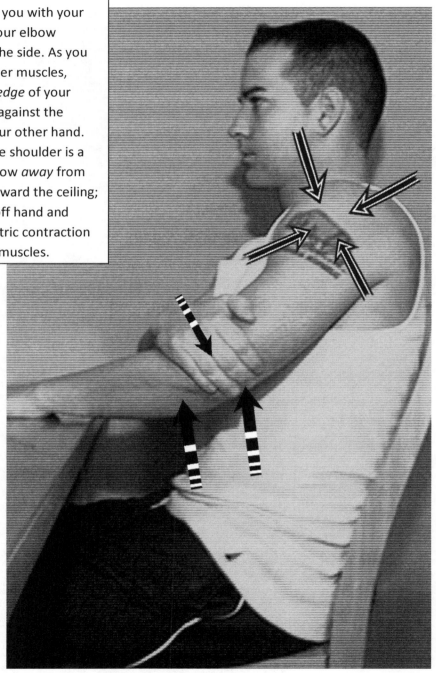

This is similar to the previous position, except that now you're leaning further forward, so you're closer to the table and your arm has more bend to it. You'll find this adjustment tends to raise your shoulder closer to your ear and thus alter the isometric contraction somewhat—engaging the back of the shoulder a bit more. Experiment with the angles and look for the best points of isometric balance or counter-tension.

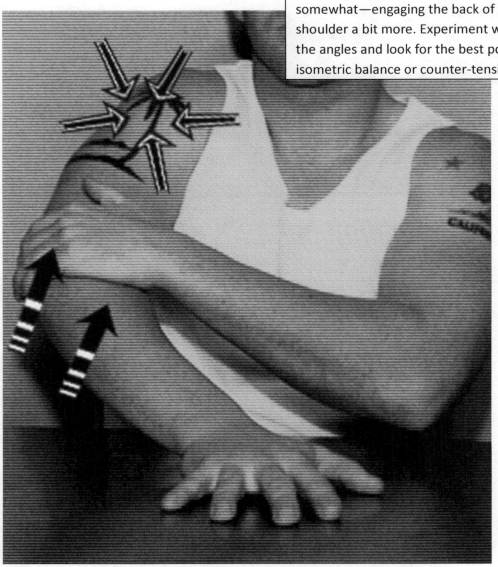

In this position, we've rotated the upper arm inward and straightened it. There is now a subtle lifting action *directly from the shoulder*; alternately, you can also pull the elbow *inward* and *downward* as you flex the shoulder isometrically—while keeping your arm straight and your palm on the table.

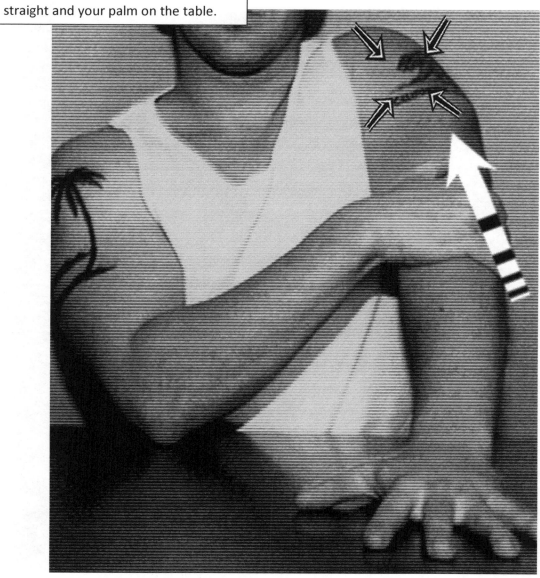

With your arm extended straight under the table, press upward against the resistance of your other hand as you flex your shoulder muscles. As an adjustment, try positioning your hand more toward the center— or off to either side. This adjustment changes the angle of engagement for the shoulder muscles as they pull the arm upward and contract.

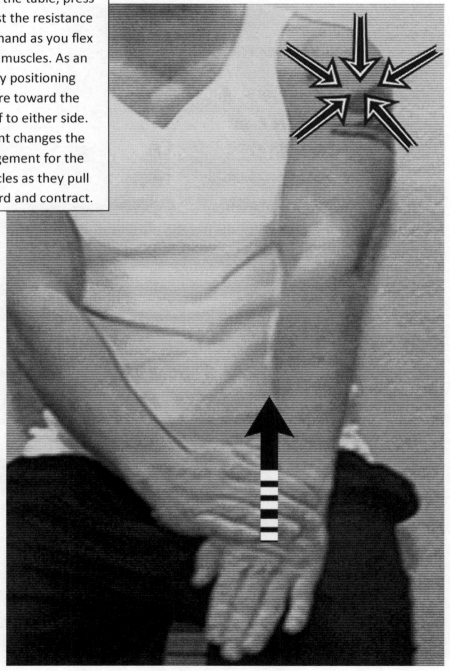

In this position you're pushing your wrist down and away as you resist with your other hand, working the shoulder muscles isometrically—especially the deltoid. Notice that whether your wrist is pulling downward, sideways or backward, you can also pull upward with your *elbow* at the same time, which involves even more of the muscles of the shoulder and intensifies the contraction. Another adjustment to this position is to sit farther back in your chair, or to flatten your palm onto your thigh.

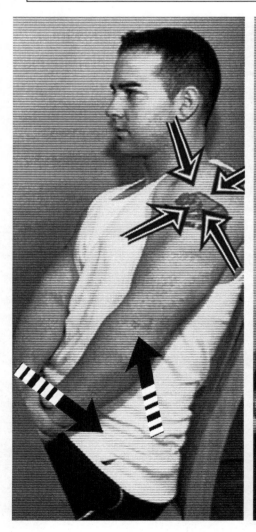
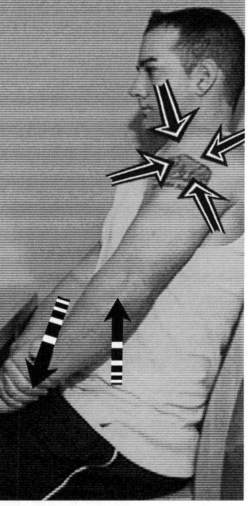

Press your hands inward against your thighs as you lift upward with your elbows, rotating the *tip of your elbow* upward toward the ceiling and flexing your shoulders. Notice that your shoulders pull *forward*; an additional adjustment to this position is to simultaneously pull the shoulders *back*, as you intensify the contraction.

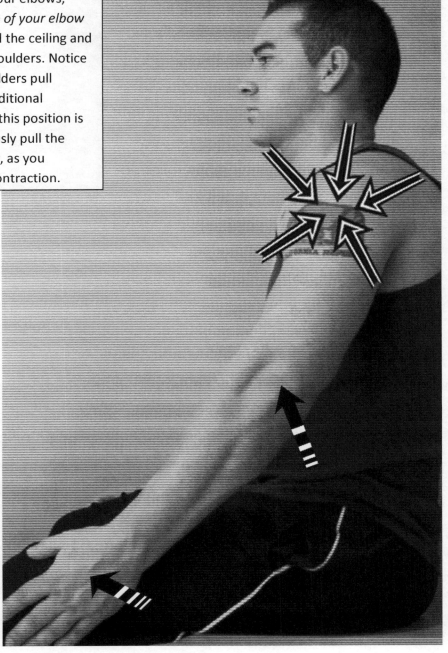

This position starts with your fists on your thighs and your elbows held slightly away from your body. Squeeze your fists strongly as you flex your shoulder muscles; without moving your arms, exert a downward and inward-pull with your elbows, while squeezing and intensely contracting the shoulder muscles.

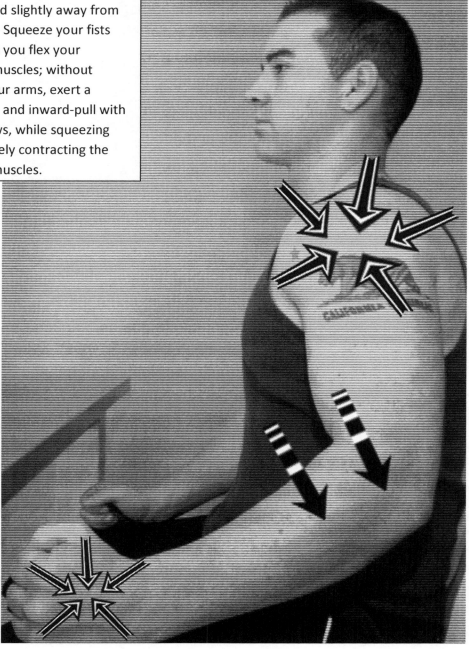

Now the fist is held lower at your side. Squeeze your fist tightly and rotate your upper arm inward as you flex the shoulder. As a balancing adjustment, pull your elbow downward and closer to your ribs, as you intensify the isometric contraction of the shoulder muscles.

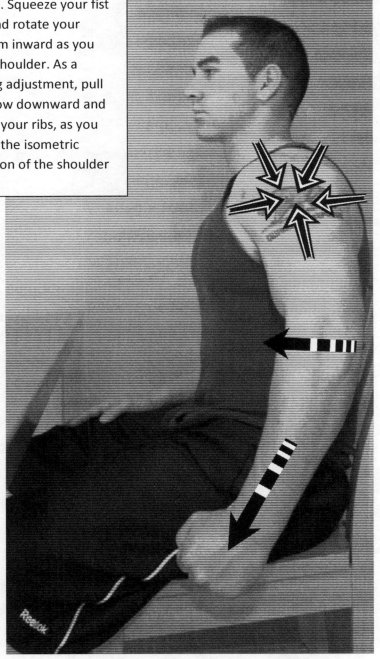

With your hands on your upper legs and your elbows pointed outward, press down onto the tops of your thighs, pushing your elbows and shoulders *forward*, and flex your shoulder muscles isometrically. As an adjustment, sit up straighter and squeeze your elbows in toward your ribs as you flex your shoulders.

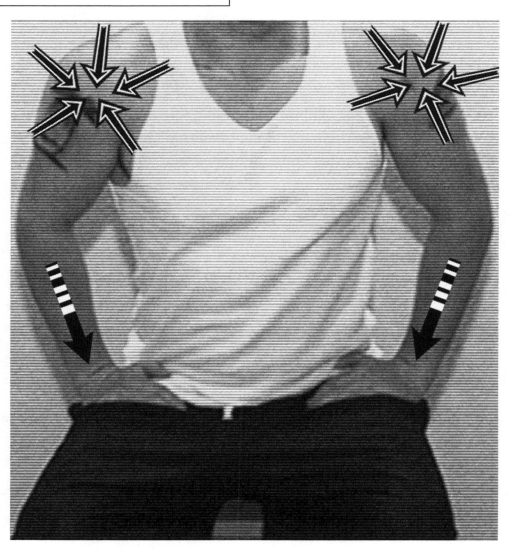

Now place your palms flat on the table with your elbows held out to the side. Flex your shoulder muscles isometrically as you pull your elbows *downward* and *inward* toward your ribs. You are engaging your shoulders here to simultaneously lift your elbows *upward* and to pull them *inward*, as you squeeze the deep shoulder muscles with isometric tension.

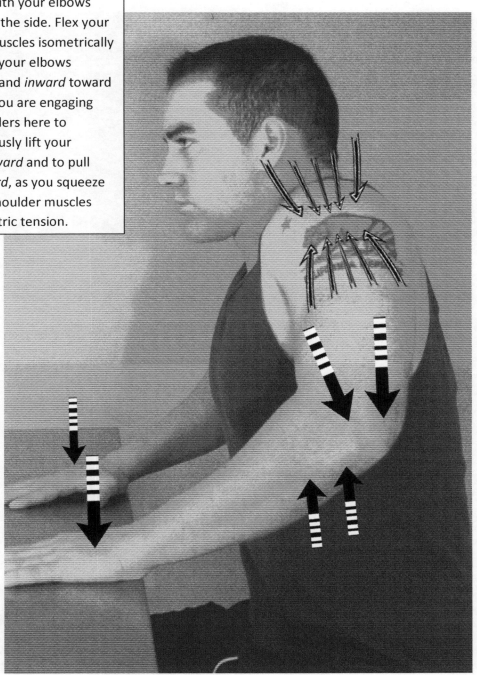

Now place your palm on your thigh, with your wrist rotated inward, so that your fingers point toward your crotch, and your elbow is pointing directly to the side. Press downward onto your thigh with your palm, and push your shoulder forward as you flex your shoulder isometrically, especially the *back* of the shoulder.

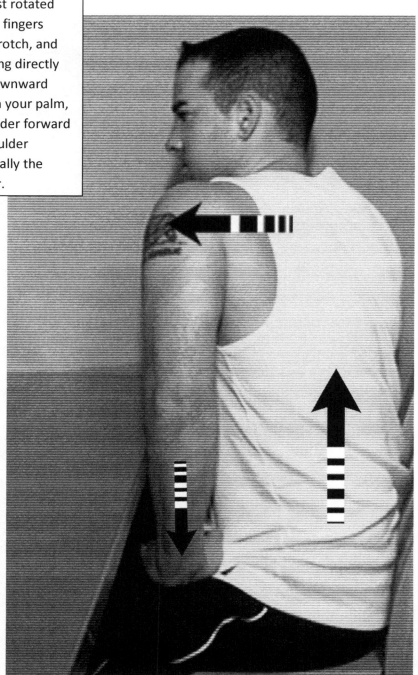

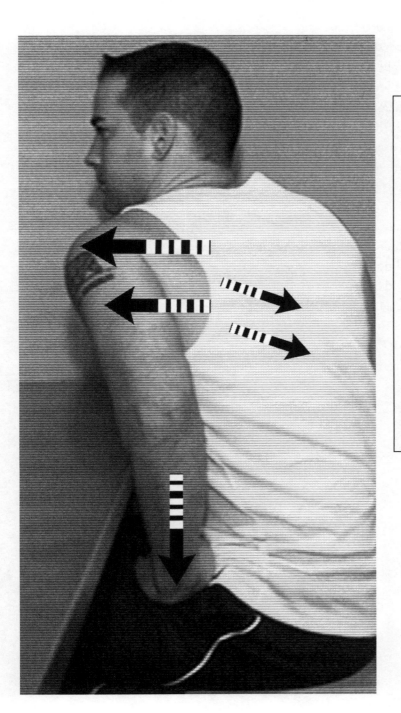

Push your shoulder forward even further now, still pressing your hand downward and flexing your shoulder muscles.

As you push your shoulder forward, pull your ribs back the other way—this exerts a pull on the *back* of your shoulder, especially the muscles under the shoulder blades and behind the deltoid; focus on flexing precisely this area.

You are simultaneously pulling your upper ribs back, *away* from your shoulder as it presses forward; let your weight sag slightly downward, as you keep your hand planted on your thigh and your elbow out to the side. Lean your torso back as you torque your shoulder forward, down and across-- this creates a stretch as well as the isometric counter-tension to really engage and flex the back of the shoulder isometrically. An additional adjustment here would be to squeeze your elbow slightly inward toward your ribs once the shoulder is fully flexed.

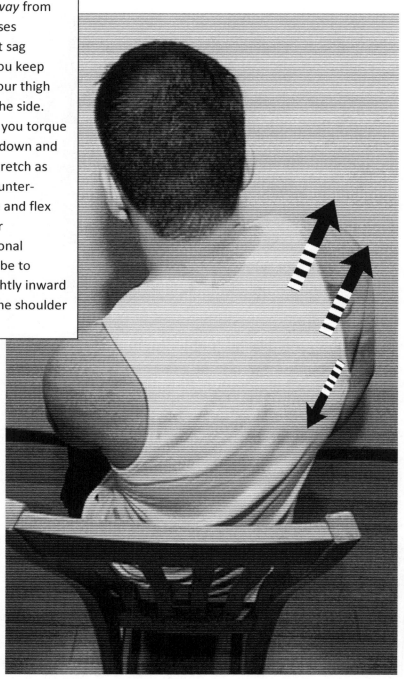

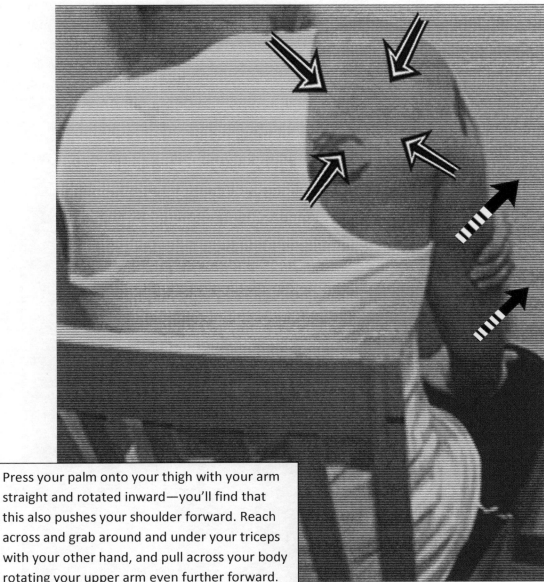

Press your palm onto your thigh with your arm straight and rotated inward—you'll find that this also pushes your shoulder forward. Reach across and grab around and under your triceps with your other hand, and pull across your body rotating your upper arm even further forward. Flex your shoulder isometrically, focusing on the back of the shoulder. It is generally good to sit up straight while using this technique; however leaning back slightly can increase the isometric tension in the shoulder.

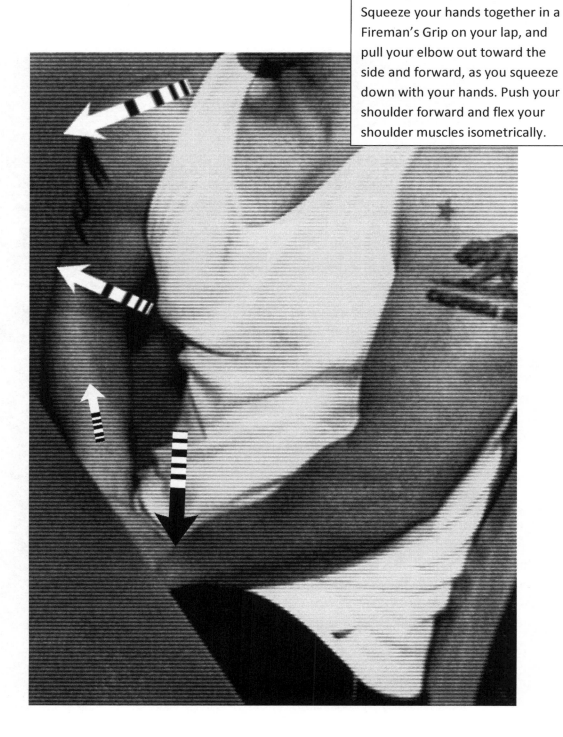

Squeeze your hands together in a Fireman's Grip on your lap, and pull your elbow out toward the side and forward, as you squeeze down with your hands. Push your shoulder forward and flex your shoulder muscles isometrically.

With your hands on the table, press your open palm against your fist; squeeze your elbow down and *in toward* your ribs as you flex your shoulder muscles isometrically.

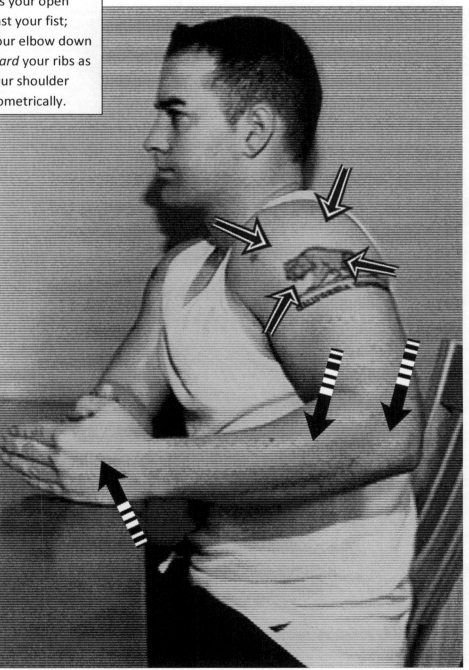

Push your palms down against your chair, and *roll your shoulders forward* by hunching them up toward your ears and pushing them forward and down. Flex your trapezius muscle, from the back of your neck along the tops of your shoulders and down between your shoulder blades.

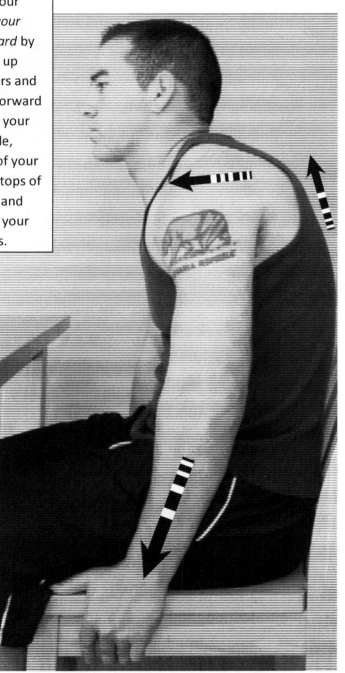

Now, grabbing *under* your chair, once again bring your shoulders up toward your ears and roll them forward; this time, however, as your shoulders push forward and flex, pull *upward* with your hands on the chair, as if you were pulling the seat of the chair off the ground. If your shoulders are properly rolled forward, you should immediately feel a strong pulling on the top of your trapezius muscle, along the back of your upper shoulders to your neck; flex the trapezius isometrically as it engages, amplifying the effect. Remember to breathe naturally, and try to find the sweet spot between *pulling up* with the hands and *pushing forward* with the shoulders, where you get the most torque on the trapezius muscle with minimal effort.

Now grip the *back* of the chair. Sit straight up, and pull your elbows and shoulders backward, keeping your arms as straight as possible. You'll feel immediately that this position engages the muscles in your shoulders and upper back, *especially* between your shoulder blades. As you pull backward with your shoulders and elbows, keeping a grip on the chair, pull your shoulder blades together behind you and flex your shoulders isometrically, focusing on the area of your trapezius in the center of your back.

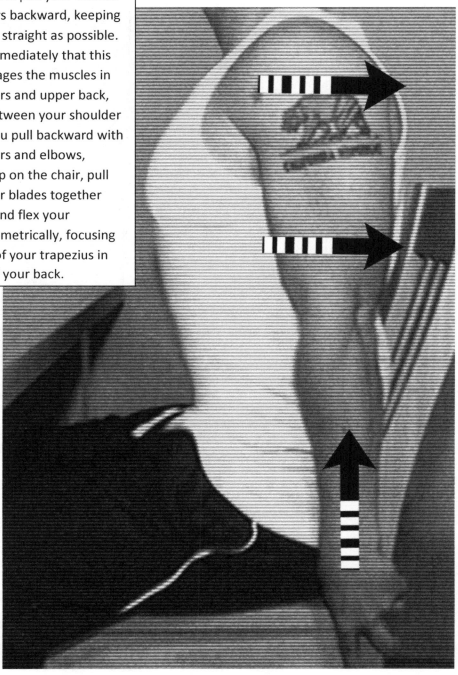

Now place your hands on your upper thighs with your fingers pointing forward. Sitting up straight, pull your elbows and shoulders directly backward, and squeeze your shoulder blades together behind you, as you flex the trapezius and the other muscles of your shoulders and upper back with isometric tension. Move your hands higher onto your thighs and push your elbows back farther behind you to intensify the contraction.

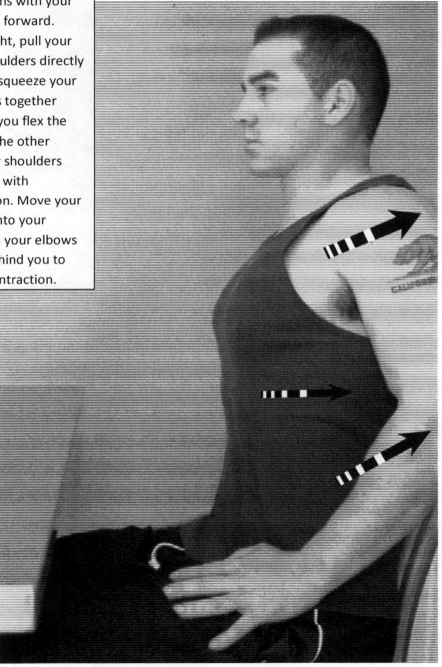

Pull your elbows and shoulders backward, and pull your shoulder blades together; notice how sitting up straighter and extending your spine upward amplifies the effect of this. Flex the shoulders with isometric contraction, working with the various counter-tensions of the shoulders—simultaneously pulling the muscles apart and pulling them together.

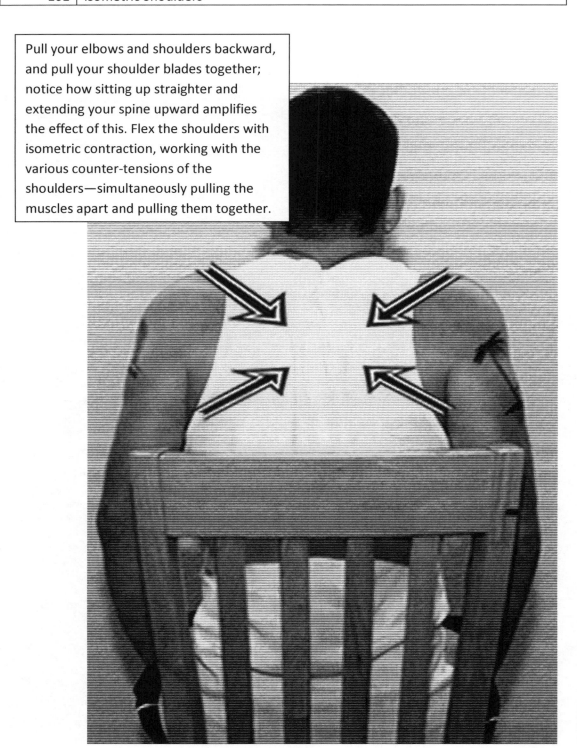

The shoulder blades squeeze together as you flex the trapezius isometrically and pull your shoulders backward. Notice how the position can be intensified by pulling the elbows towards each other behind the back, or by leaning forward.

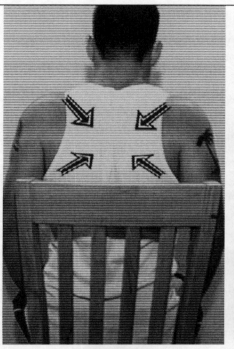
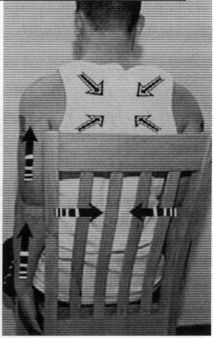
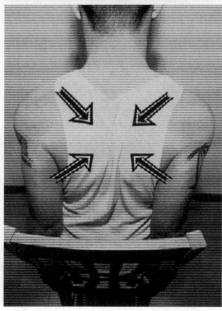
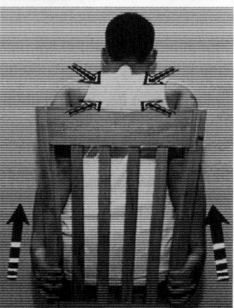

Here you're leaning back, in a confident and casual stretching position. Pull your elbows back and toward one another behind you, your shoulder blades pulling closer together as you flex and contract the entire upper shoulders and the trapezius with isometric tension. As an additional adjustment you can lean back further and push your chest forward—this has the added effect of opening up and stretching your chest as you work on the backs of the shoulders.

This is similar to the previous position, except that now you're sitting up straight instead of leaning back. Notice that your hands are braced against your head, so if you push your head back into your hands you generate additional isometric resistance against your shoulder muscles, which are pulling your elbows back. Again, look for the *sweet spots of isometric equilibrium,* which allow you to engage your muscles with minimum effort and maximum effect. Don't practice this position if you have neck problems or soreness. Remember to breathe, keep your face relaxed, and don't strain.

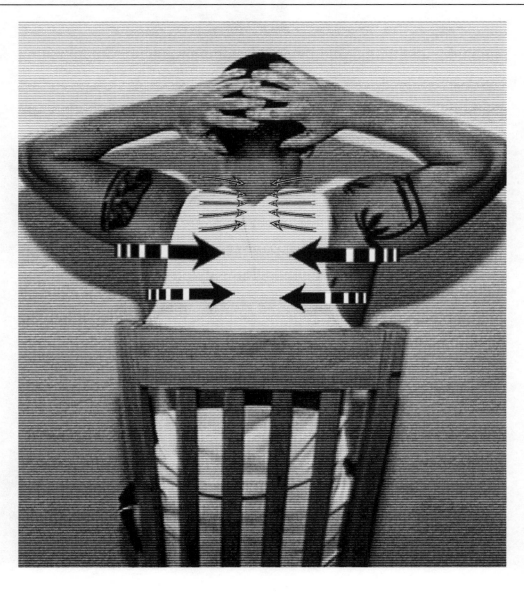

Here's your standard card protector position combined with an isometric shoulder contraction. Simultaneously push your hand downward and lift your elbow upward, as you squeeze and flex your shoulder muscles isometrically. An intense, focused isometric contraction from a stationary position can actually work your shoulder muscles more intensely than calisthenics or lifting weights—*without* any wear and tear on the cartilage, tendons or ligaments.

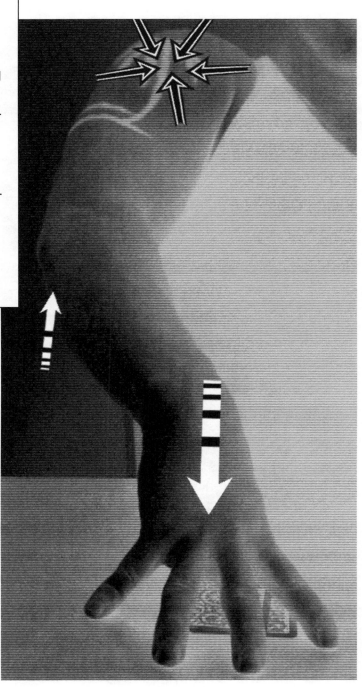

Isometric Back

The muscles of the back are among the most powerful in the entire body. The lattissimus dorsi run along both sides of the body from the shoulders to the waist and form the well-known V-shape. The trapezius muscle is the large diamond shaped muscle extending from the neck down between the shoulders to the middle of the back. Additionally, there are many smaller back muscles, including the multifidus and erector spinae muscles, which surround and connect the spine, shoulders, ribs, abdomen and pelvis. Some of these muscles even extend down through the pelvis and connect to the upper thigh.

When practicing isometrics we will often focus on the latissimus dorsi muscles, or "lats", because these muscles are functionally very prominent and are readily engaged using isometric technique. However, keep in mind that when you engage your lats, you often also engage other back muscles to some degree as well. Sometimes you'll want to want try to flex the lats in isolation as much as possible, while at other times you'll want to involve the various other muscles of the back and spine and work them together in synergy with the lats. In some isometric techniques, we will shift the focus to the muscles of the central back completely—flexing and squeezing the muscles surrounding the spine with isometric force, engaging and extending your backbone like a powerful steel spring.

Allow yourself to *feel* the muscles of the back; get in touch with how your back works; understand it. Think about your posture and make an effort to control and activate the muscles around your spine, which you may have taken largely for granted up until now.

When you work your back muscles effectively, you get a definite "pump", and the pleasant oxygenated feeling is even more pleasurable because of the presence and proximity of so many large nerves in the back. Also when you do back isometrics, think about the idea of "opening" your back, by which I mean opening the flow of blood in and around the spine, as well as taking pressure off the spinal disks and nerves and allowing a smoother flow of cerebrospinal fluid within the spinal column itself. Extending the back, flexing, and working the muscles in and around the spine will increase blood flow to those areas and allow you straighten out various kinks caused by tension, lethargy and bad posture. It all starts with getting in touch with your back muscles and getting a feel for engaging them directly using isometric technique. Remember to relax the back, also. Flex, contract and then relax: the ability to flex the back and the spine increases your ability to release and relax it as well, and makes it all the more sweeter when you do.

Leaning forward, reach between your legs and grab under your thighs with both hands. With straight arms and a firm grip, pull upward against your legs using your back muscles, flexing your back isometrically. Work the lat muscles, under the arms, as shown.

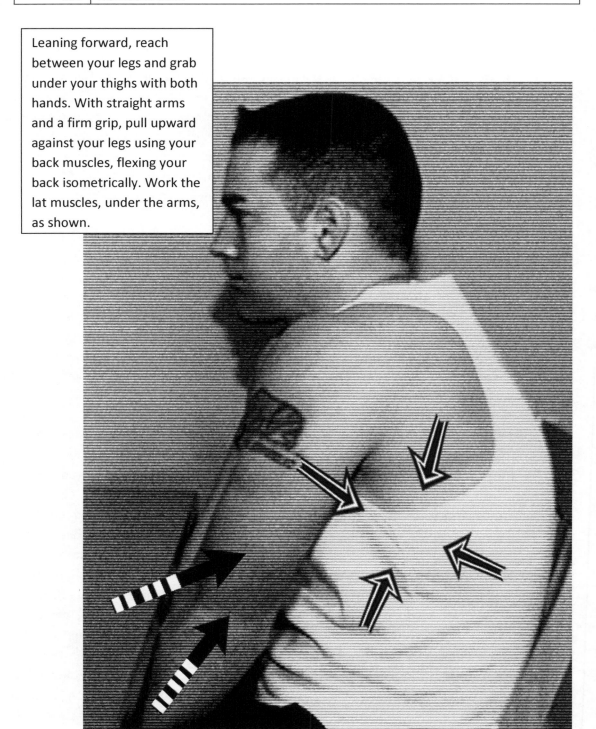

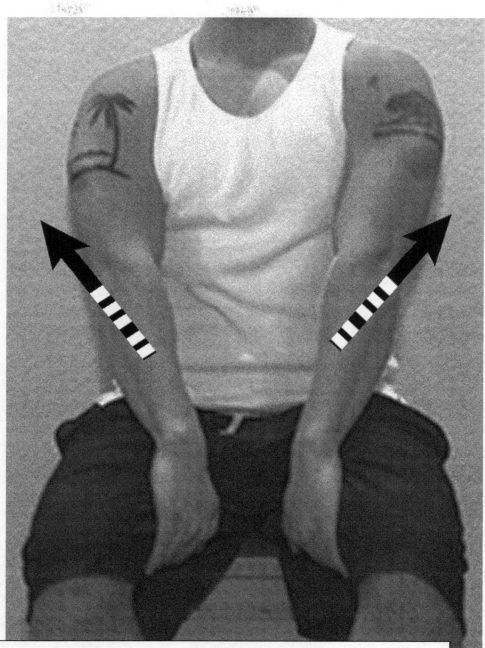

Here's the same position from a different perspective. Notice that this time we're pulling up and slightly *outward*, whereas in the previous technique we were pulling the elbows slightly *inward*, toward the ribs. You want to feel the muscles of the back spreading and flexing from the spine; remember to breathe naturally.

Here again you're grabbing the undersides of your thighs with your hands; but this time your arms are bent—your elbows stick out sideways. Pull upwards as you widen your elbows and flex the lat muscles isometrically. Sit up straighter and extend your spine upward to increase the pull on your back

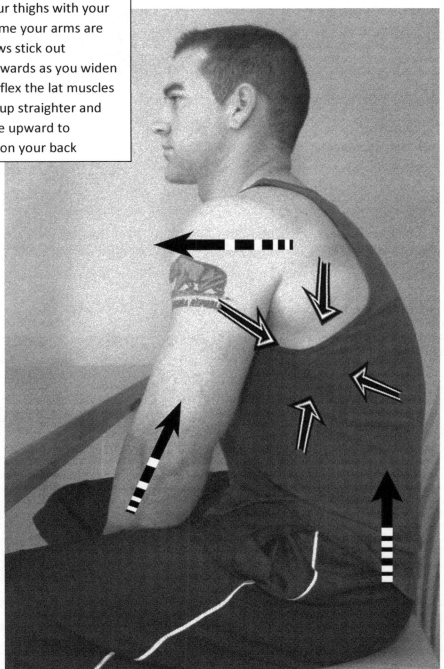

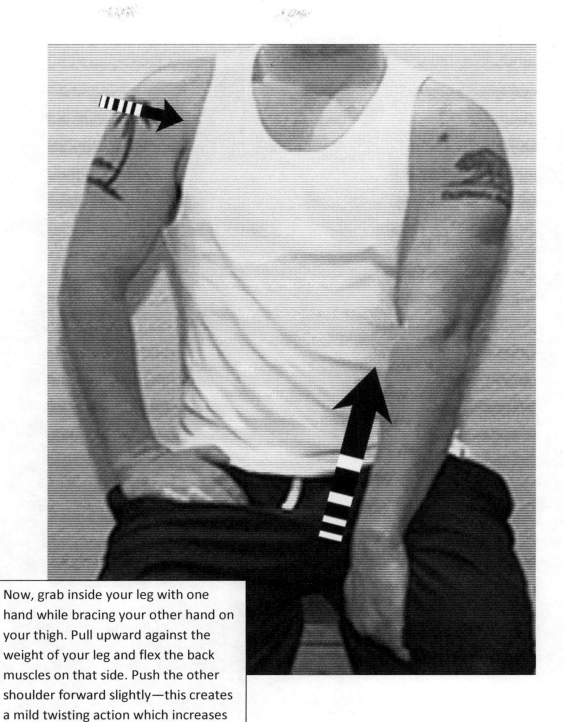

Now, grab inside your leg with one hand while bracing your other hand on your thigh. Pull upward against the weight of your leg and flex the back muscles on that side. Push the other shoulder forward slightly—this creates a mild twisting action which increases the isometric tension.

Grab inside your thigh with one hand, and grab the back of your chair with the other hand. Pull upward against your leg, flexing your lat muscle on that side as you push your shoulder across your body, twisting forward. Straighten up through your spine, sitting with erect posture. With your body twisted forward you are pulling directly upward with the lat muscle, as you squeeze and contract it isometrically.

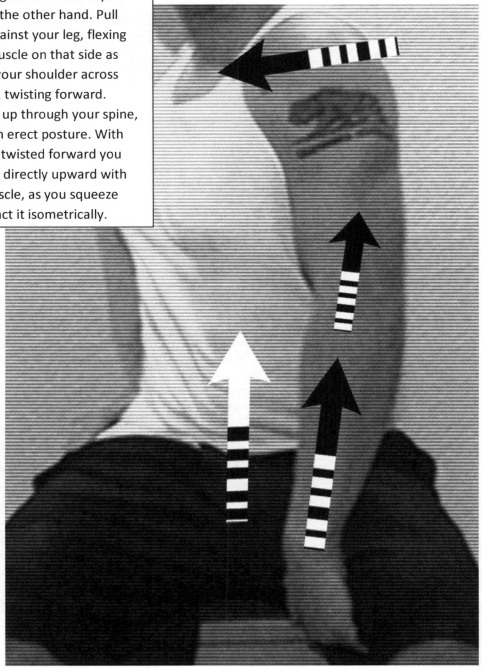

Now, grab around the front of your knees with both hands. Pull upwards against your knees as you contract your back muscles isometrically. Feel the muscles of your back squeezing together toward your spine as you sit up straighter and push your chest forward. In this technique you are rotating your upper arms outward—your inner elbows face upward and you are pulling *in* towards your body as you flex the back.

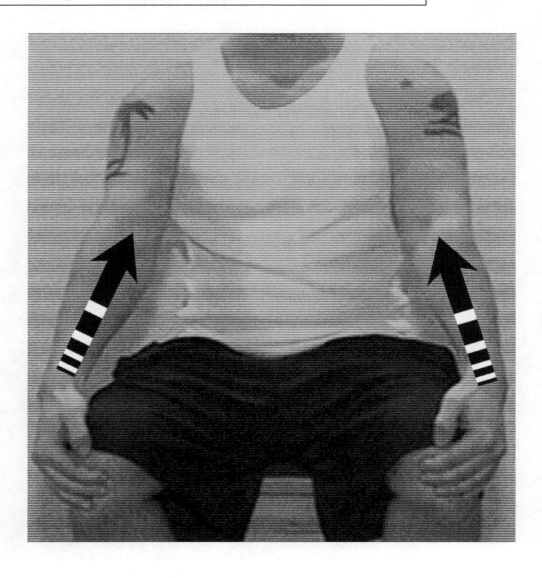

In this technique you are again grabbing around the outsides of your knees and pulling against your legs; this time however your upper arms are rotated more inward—and your angle of pull is straight up toward your shoulders. Your back muscles are flexed isometrically, the two halves of your body pulling together from your lats to your spine as you sit upward. Let the isometric contraction of your back muscles be the primary thing—the flexing of the muscles pulls your arms toward you, and *not* the other way around.

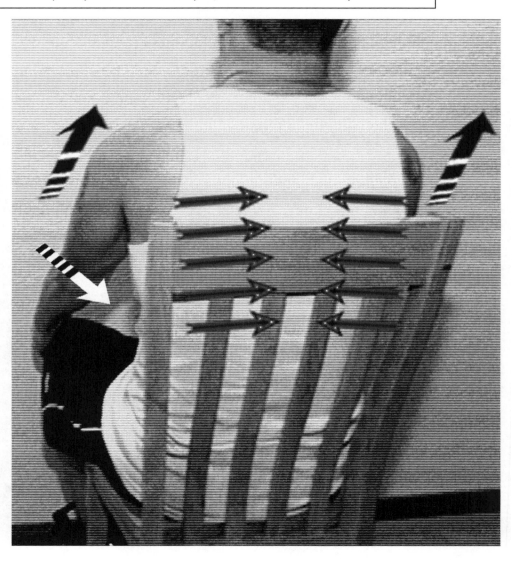

Now grip the front of your knee with one hand, while bracing your other hand on your upper thigh. Pull upward from your back muscles, flexing them with isometric tension. Squeeze and hold the isometric contraction, isolating the latissimus dorsi area under your arm.

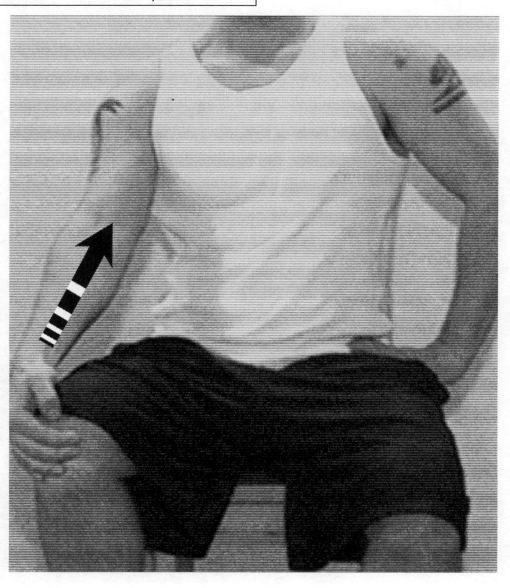

Now grab the *outside* of your thigh, gripping either your pants or your outer hamstring tendon, whichever is easiest. Your arm is bent, and you pull your elbow upward and inward, toward your ribs, as you flex the lat muscles on that side. Pull your elbow in *sideways*, in to your ribs, and really put the isometric squeeze on those back muscles.

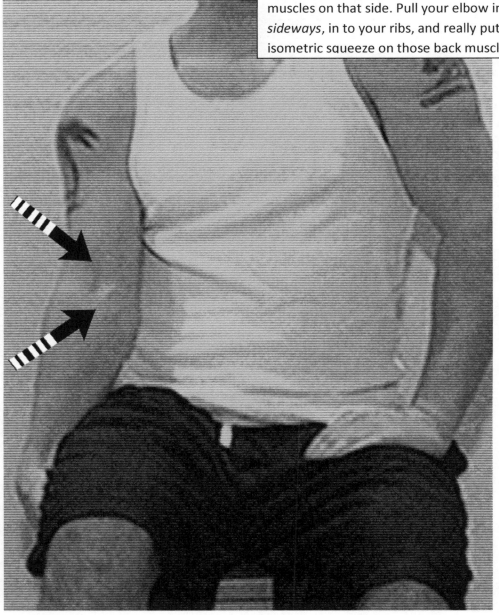

Now grab under your chair with both hands. Pull upward, as you push your shoulders and elbows forward, flexing and *spreading* your back muscles outward from your spine. The lat muscles in particular spread outward under your arms, forming a 'V' shape. Sit up straight, and continue to pull upward with your hands to increase the flex of the lats.

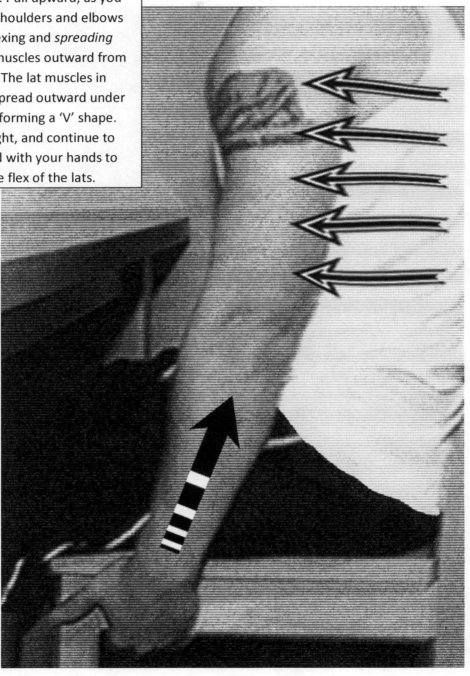

Place your fists on your upper thighs and, keeping your arms close to your ribs, pull both of your elbows straight back as you squeeze and flex the back muscles with isometric contraction. Sit up straight and try to flex the spinal erector muscles in the middle of your back. Visualize your spinal column as a coil of solid steel— activate and flex the muscles surrounding your spine. Be sure to breathe normally while you're flexed; and afterwards, be sure to release and relax your back muscles.

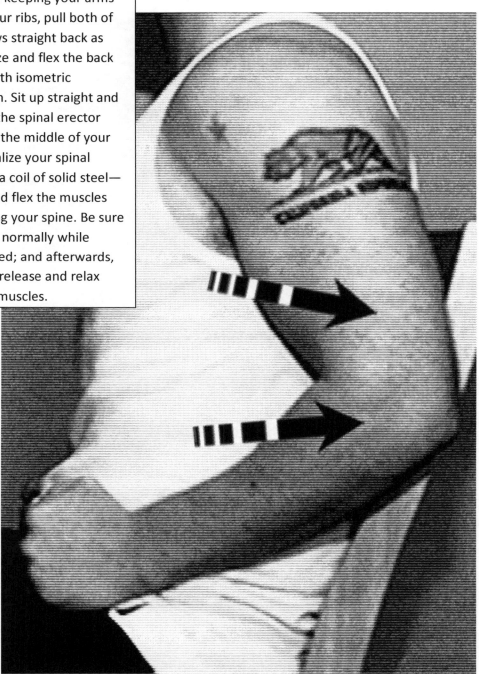

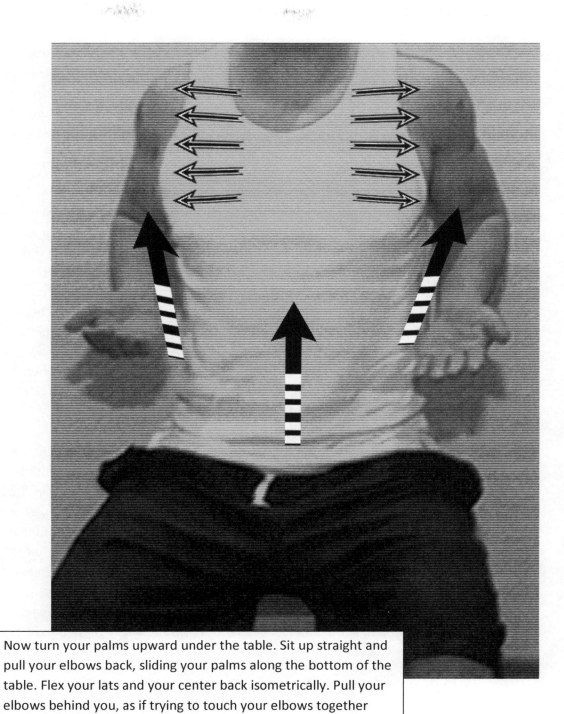

Now turn your palms upward under the table. Sit up straight and pull your elbows back, sliding your palms along the bottom of the table. Flex your lats and your center back isometrically. Pull your elbows behind you, as if trying to touch your elbows together behind your back. Breathe.

Isometric Neck

Wrestlers and fighters are well aware that a strong neck is very crucial for toughness and figthing ability; strengthening the muscles of the neck also helps to alleviate and prevent neck aches and neck pain, which can be caused by poor posture and excessive muscular tension stored in the neck. Working the muscles of the neck can also help prevent the buildup of arterial plaque in the carotids, and also improves your appearance by strenghtening your jaw line and reducing double chins.

Poker players often lean their heads against their hands in various positions, so using isometrics to strengthen the neck while playing poker is easy. As always, be sure to keep your face relaxed and to not overstrain, *especially* when you are working your neck. Never overdo it. Don't twist your neck or force it in any way. Use passive resistance with one of your hands and smoothly press your head against this resistance with your neck muscles, from a fixed position. When you practice isometrics to strenghten your neck use moderation. Focus, relaxation and the mind-body connection is really crucial here. Just tilt or press your head slightly against the resistance of your hand, and as you feel the muscles engage flex them smoothly without straining, remembering to breathe naturally, then relax the muscles and let go of the tension in the neck. As you become more aware of both flexing and relaxing your neck you'll notice the tendency to store tension there, and how much better you feel when you get rid of that tension.

At the poker table, you have opportunities to use neck isometrics when you lean back and stretch, when you rest your forehead against your palm or when you cover your face with your hands. It fairly common for a poker player to play with or fondle his or her head at times.These natural fidgety moments provide a good opportunity to *sneakily* get in some quick neck isometrics. In fact, you no doubt do something similar without even thinking about it on occasion, yawning or stretching your neck one way or the other after sitting at the table for a long time; however now we're doing it in a much more deliberate, focused manner and consciously using proper isometric technique. In this chapter we show the head pushing forward, to the side and to the back, with the most basic and direct hand positioning. Feel free to interpolate between the angles and directions of pressure, and to innovate with the hand positions—whatever feels and looks natural to you is good.

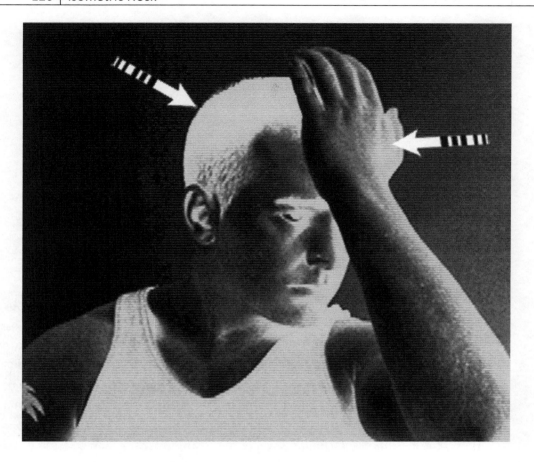

Place your hand on your forehead and flex your neck muscles as you press your forehead into your palm. Resist and push back with your hand. Focus on the contraction of the neck muscles, especially the two ridges of muscle on the *back* of your neck that extend upward from the trapezius. Try pushing your chin slightly outward as you flex. Remember to breathe, and don't over-strain. Be sure to keep your face relaxed when working the neck, and be sure to relax the muscles of the neck after flexing them. Notice that this is a very easy position to practice while playing poker, as many players will place an elbow on the table and rest their forehead on their palm during game play.

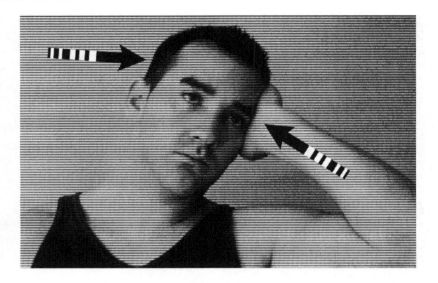

Here are a couple of additional neck-flex variations: Above, lean the side of your head onto your hand, presumably with your elbow resting on the table, and press your head against your hand as you flex the side of your neck. Below, clasp your hands behind your head and lean back in the classic boss pose; with your elbows pointed forward and your arms relaxed, gently push your head back into your hands as you flex the neck muscles. Be sure to breathe normally and *do not* over-strain. Make a conscious effort to release and relax the muscles of your neck after you finish; these isometric techniques will burn off stored tension and stress in your neck muscles, so be sure to let yourself relax afterwards to take full advantage of this.

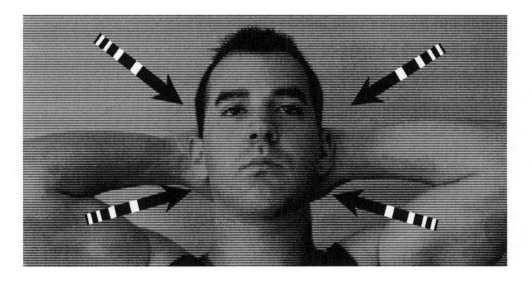

Isometric Thighs

The muscles of the thigh are the hamstrings and the quadriceps. The quadriceps, or quads as they called, are on the front of the leg and serve to extend the knee and straighten the leg. The hamstrings are the rear muscles of the thigh and serve to flex the knee and bend the leg. In this sense, the quads and hamstrings are an antagonistic pair with a relationship similar to that of the biceps and triceps.

The Hamstrings

The hamstrings are large muscles and very powerful, and from a seated position we have to use isometrics in a very specific way and proceed with caution. With your leg completely bent, if you strongly flex your hamstring the muscle can cramp up—pulling together with surprising power. Because the leg is fully bent there's no balancing counter-force against the contraction of the hamstring muscle, and the hamstrings are so powerful that the contraction can cause the leg to seize together into a ball of muscle, which is painful and difficult to unbend. The point here is that we don't fully flex the hamstring muscle with the leg completely bent; we have to approach it with a bit of caution.

We either work with the leg partially bent, bracing it open with the opposite leg, or we keep the leg straight, actively stretching and *extending* the leg lengthwise as we flex the hamstrings isometrically. To get an idea of this action, imagine from a sitting position extending your leg outward through the foot, lengthening the leg as if someone were under the table pulling your foot as you contract the hamstring isometrically.

These two actions, extending the leg and contracting the hamstring, counter-balance each other. Sometimes you'll be able to do them simultaneously, and sometimes you'll subtly alternate between them. Try and find the sweet spots, or points of balanced tension, that will allow you to hold and sustain the isometric hamstring contraction and really work the muscles effectively. Afterwards, really let go and *relax* the hamstrings; breathe into them and let them completely relax. You might even massage your thigh for moment. The hamstrings are a muscle where tension can get stored, and long term this can affect your lower back, your posture and even your moods. Burning off some of that extra tension in your hamstrings, while at the same time learning to relax them, is a very good thing— especially if you're spending a lot of time sitting at the poker table.

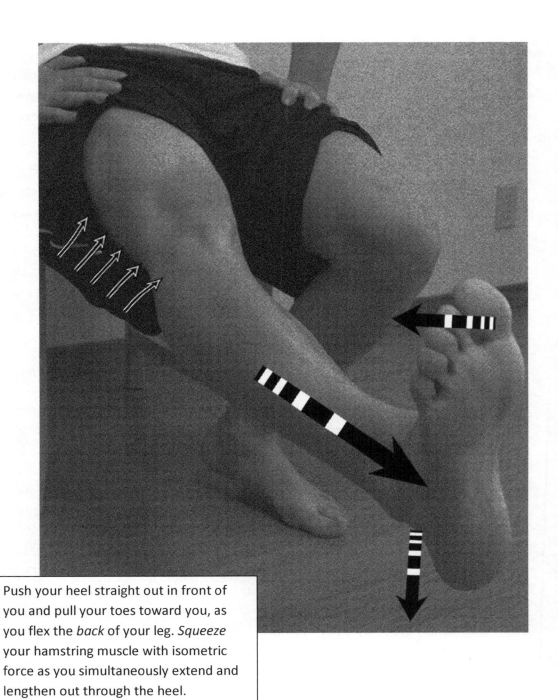

Push your heel straight out in front of you and pull your toes toward you, as you flex the *back* of your leg. *Squeeze* your hamstring muscle with isometric force as you simultaneously extend and lengthen out through the heel.

Look closely at the above illustration, and notice a few things:

- The hamstring muscle is fully flexed.
- The leg is extended straight, but the straightening of the leg does not force against the knee joint. Rather, the true extension of the leg has a *lengthening* action.
- The contraction of the hamstring exerts pull on the heel to come back toward the thigh—to bend the leg.
- One counter-force to the hamstring contraction is the extension of the leg.
- The other counter-force to the hamstring contraction is the pulling back of the toes. When the toes pull back toward the knee, it stretches the hamstrings: with the hamstrings stretched, isometric contraction is even more effective; not only will your muscles not cramp, but your flexibility will improve also.

Experiment with these isometric polarities and counter-tensions; what you're looking for is a balance between strongly flexing the hamstring and extending the leg; the hamstring pulling upward behind the leg, while the leg pushes straight outward.

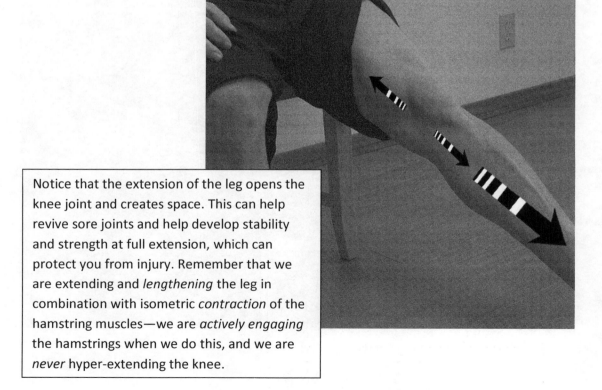

Notice that the extension of the leg opens the knee joint and creates space. This can help revive sore joints and help develop stability and strength at full extension, which can protect you from injury. Remember that we are extending and *lengthening* the leg in combination with isometric *contraction* of the hamstring muscles—we are *actively engaging* the hamstrings when we do this, and we are *never* hyper-extending the knee.

Flexing your hamstring isometrically, pull your foot inward, bending your leg. Your other leg, positioned inside, resists it by pushing outward; bracing it by placing the resisting foot on the floor gives you more leverage. Focus the isometric contraction in the hamstring muscle.

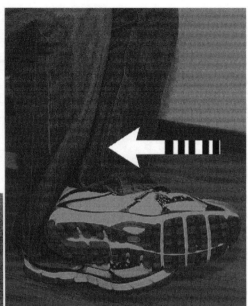

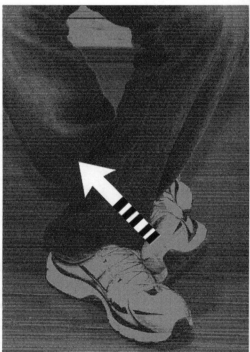

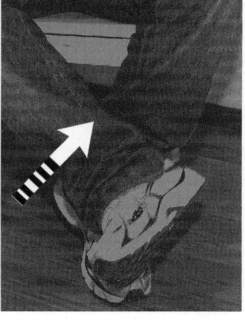

This technique is extremely good for working off excess adrenaline or stress; try it if you feel yourself becoming tilted. Be sure to let your hamstrings relax afterward and stretch or extend your leg.

The Quadriceps

The quadriceps extends the knee and straightens the leg. When you're running, jumping, kicking or even standing your quadriceps muscles come into play. The thighbone—the femur—is known to be the largest bone in the human body, and the quadriceps are easily one of the strongest and largest muscles. Working the quads increases the production of testosterone, speeds up your metabolism, builds muscle, and burns fat.

Because the quads extend the knee, they can't easily be over-contracted, so we can use isometrics on them with either a straight or a bent leg. From a sitting position, pressing one or both feet into the ground while flexing the quads, kind of like doing a leg press machine at the gym, is very effective. The kind of deep muscle work generated by pushing downward, with the legs bent at a 90 degree angle, combined with proper isometric technique, will quickly kick-start your metabolism and get your thighs feeling pumped.

Using isometrics to work the quads with a straight leg is also very effective. Flexing the quadriceps extends the knee, and when your leg is straight the isometric contraction of the quads on the front of the thigh *lifts* the kneecap. Ideally we want to think about extending the entire leg and lengthening it as we flex the quadriceps—so while the kneecap pulls upward we are also pushing out through the foot. This is true whether we are pulling the toes back and pushing through our heel, or whether we are pushing through the ball of the foot. There are differences between pushing through the heel or the ball of the foot when working the quads isometrically. With the foot *flexed* and the toes pulled back, the isometric contraction of the quadriceps tends to *pull the toes farther back* toward the knee; with the ball of the foot extended, the action of the quads tends to also involve the rear of the calf and pull the *heel* back farther. Experiment with both of these positions and try some variations and in-between positions; see if you can isolate the actions of the muscles and see how they work. Think about not only flexing the quadriceps, but also opening and strengthening the knee joint as well as the entire front of the leg.

When working on the quads, mentally focusing and really *feeling* what's going on *inside* the muscle is vital. We're really taking muscle control to the next level here and we're getting in touch with our *lower body*. As always, releasing and relaxing your muscles after an extended contraction is essential, and feels great. When your upper-thighs are really pumped from isometrics, and when you deeply relax them, you may feel a surge of warmth or sexual energy in your crotch. This is in part from increased blood flow and oxygenation in the area, as well as the release of stored tension in the upper thighs and pelvis.

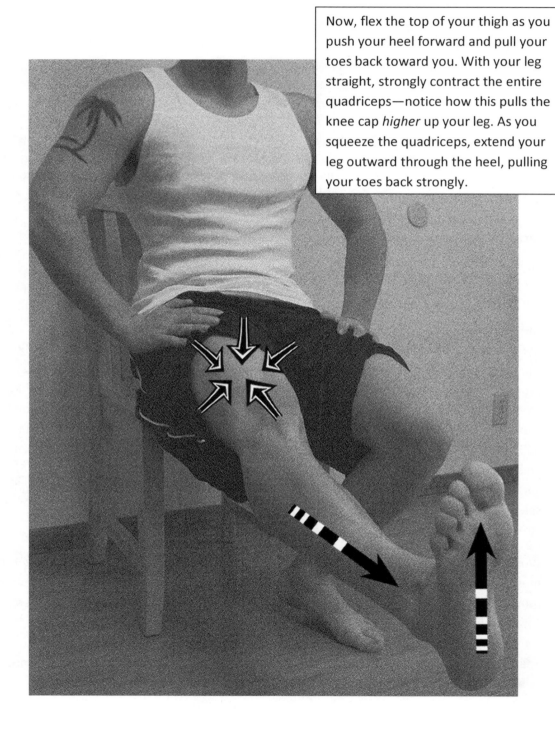

Now, flex the top of your thigh as you push your heel forward and pull your toes back toward you. With your leg straight, strongly contract the entire quadriceps—notice how this pulls the knee cap *higher* up your leg. As you squeeze the quadriceps, extend your leg outward through the heel, pulling your toes back strongly.

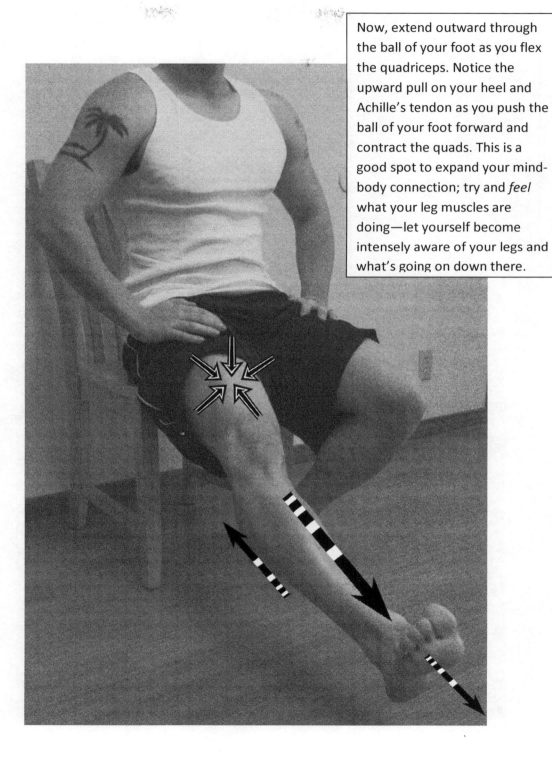

Now, extend outward through the ball of your foot as you flex the quadriceps. Notice the upward pull on your heel and Achille's tendon as you push the ball of your foot forward and contract the quads. This is a good spot to expand your mind-body connection; try and *feel* what your leg muscles are doing—let yourself become intensely aware of your legs and what's going on down there.

With your leg straight and your heel on the ground, contract your quadriceps isometrically, pulling your knee cap upward as you extend your leg through your ankle and heel. Do *not* hyper-extend your knee; in fact, partially bending your knee and also involving the hamstring muscle in the isometric contraction can be a useful adjustment.

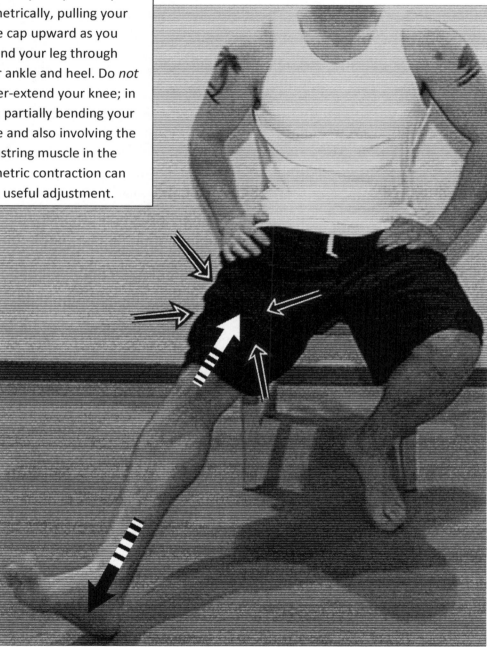

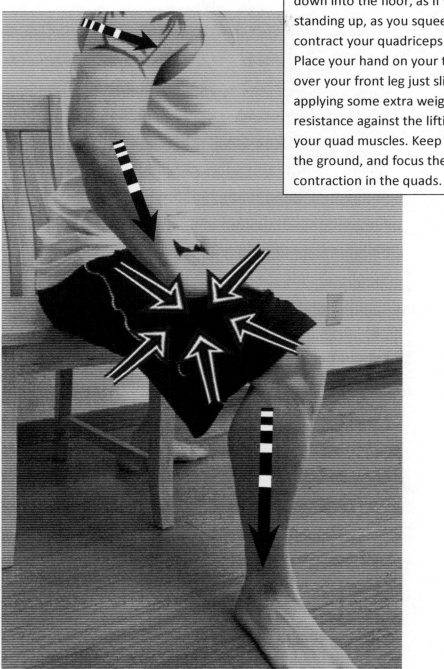

From a sitting position, press one foot down into the floor, as if you were standing up, as you squeeze and contract your quadriceps isometrically. Place your hand on your thigh and lean over your front leg just slightly, applying some extra weight and resistance against the lifting action of your quad muscles. Keep your heel on the ground, and focus the isometric contraction in the quads.

Sitting up straight with both hands on your thighs, press your feet into the ground and flex your quadriceps with firm isometric contraction. Accelerate *smoothly* into the contraction, remembering to breathe naturally as you hold it and squeeze your quads. After each contraction, really *let go* and relax your thigh muscles—this combination of isometrics and relaxation for the thighs is an *incredible* stress reliever, and can really help you stay grounded. Working your thighs burns stored tension and stress, and can also significantly increase your testosterone levels.

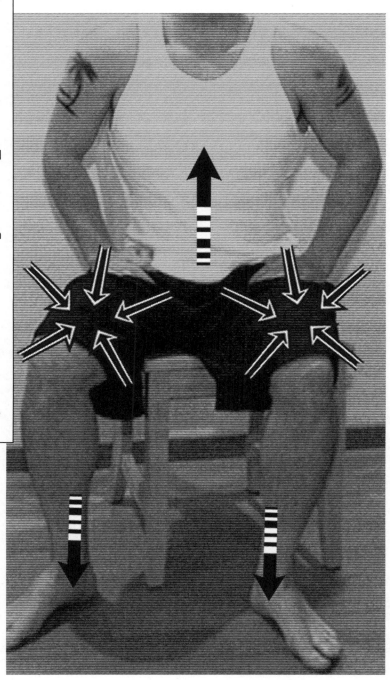

Isometric Calves

For simplicity's sake, we'll describe the calf muscles in terms of the front and the back of the calf. Along the outer-front region of your lower leg there is a ridge of muscle next to the shinbone, and extending from your knee to your ankle. The back and inner area of your calf consist of muscles extending from the Achilles' tendon to the back of the knee.

The action of the rear calf muscles, when flexed, can be described as pushing the top of the foot down away from the knee, or more accurately pulling the heel *upward* toward the back of the knee. The contraction of the back of the calf pulls on the Achilles' tendon and thus lifts the heel—crucial in such fundamental actions as walking. We could also describe this action of the back of the calf as pointing the toe, pushing out the ball of the foot, or in terms of calisthenics or weightlifting *raising* the calf and lifting through the ball of the foot. When we contract the back of the calf isometrically, the action pulls the heel upward, pushes the top and ball of the foot downward, and pulls the calf muscle higher on the leg.

The front muscle of the calf, the tibialis anterior, essentially forms an antagonistic pair with the rear muscles of the calf. The action of the front calf muscle is the opposite of the rear: it lifts the foot, pulling the toes upward toward the knee. Additionally, it stabilizes the ankle, and functionally this interplay of the front and back calf muscles is integral to standing, walking, jumping, dancing and agility of all sorts.

The front muscle of the calf tends to be the more neglected of the two, since the back muscles of the calf are larger and more impressive looking. They can also be worked out more easily with exercises such as standard calf-raises. It takes more effort to effectively target and contract the *front* muscles of the calves—lifting up onto the ball of your foot seems to be a more natural, common action than pulling the toes upward toward the shins, so isolating the front of the calves tends to be more difficult. The development of the front of the calves is essential, however, for true combat-ready strength: it toughens the front of the leg and it increases balance and stability. Experiment with turning your foot inward or outward and see how that affects the contraction of the front of the calf. Focus on controlling and flexing the front of the ankle as well—keeping the foot alive and engaged. Also, experiment with lifting up through the *inside* of your ankle to your knee, whether you're working the front of the calf, the rear of the calf, or both sides simultaneously. This action adds torsion to the contraction of the calf muscles and works to align the ankle with the knee, and strengthen the more delicate inner area of the ankle.

Turning your leg outward, press the ball of your foot into the floor and flex your calf muscle. Lift upward through the *inside* of your ankle, as you strongly contract the back of your calf isometrically.

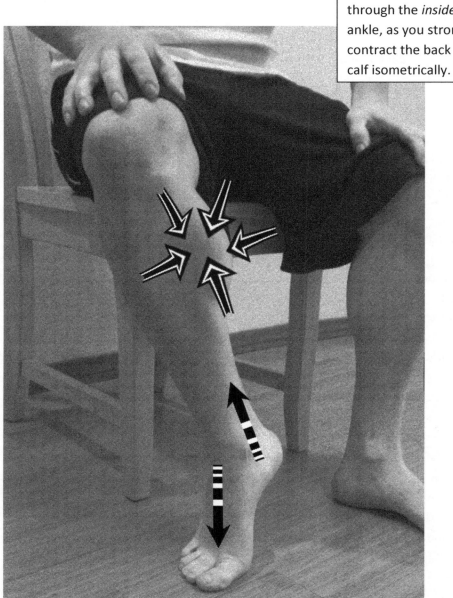

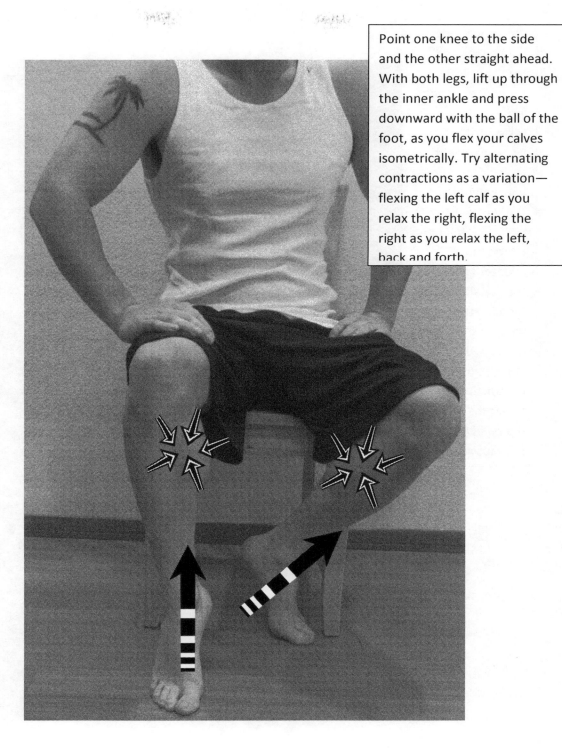

Point one knee to the side and the other straight ahead. With both legs, lift up through the inner ankle and press downward with the ball of the foot, as you flex your calves isometrically. Try alternating contractions as a variation—flexing the left calf as you relax the right, flexing the right as you relax the left, back and forth.

Put your hands on your knees and lean your weight forward onto your legs—adding resistance as you lift upward with your calves. Flex your calves hard at the top of the calf-raise, and hold the contraction. Squeeze. Notice that by altering the tilt and angle of your foot you can direct and focus the isometric contraction to either the *inside* or the *outside* of the calf muscles.

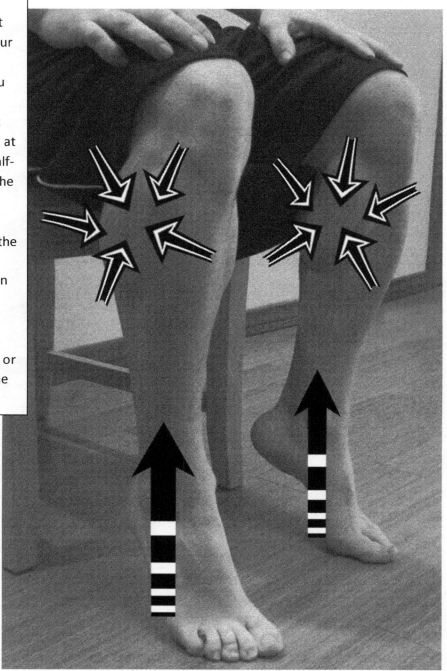

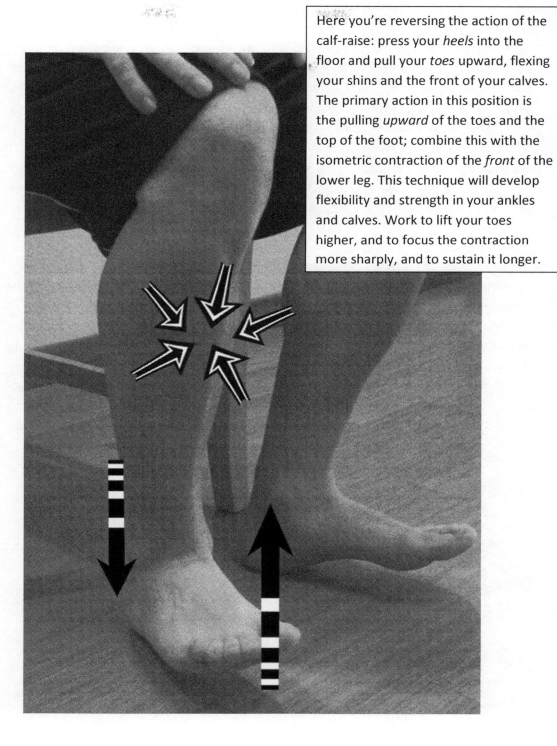

Here you're reversing the action of the calf-raise: press your *heels* into the floor and pull your *toes* upward, flexing your shins and the front of your calves. The primary action in this position is the pulling *upward* of the toes and the top of the foot; combine this with the isometric contraction of the *front* of the lower leg. This technique will develop flexibility and strength in your ankles and calves. Work to lift your toes higher, and to focus the contraction more sharply, and to sustain it longer.

Isometric Hips and Butt

The muscles of the hips and butt connect with the femurs, the pelvis, the spine, as well as the muscles of the lower back, thighs and abdomen. Besides the gluteus maximus, which most people are familiar with, there are also many other muscles in the hip region, including many small muscles that run through and around the pelvis and interact in very complex ways. When we use isometrics to work the hips and butt, these internal muscles *will* tend to get activated, and you should be aware of flexing and relaxing the deeper structures of the hips and pelvis. In terms of functional isometrics, however, we're going to focus on closing the hips inward, which works the inner groin region, opening the hips outward, which works the sides of the hips, and isometrically contracting the gluteus maximus or butt muscles.

When working with the opening or closing action of the hips we can use resistance from the hands to engage the muscles in-place, and then amplify the muscular contraction using isometrics; or we can work these muscles *without* using resistance from the hands, opening and closing the hips simultaneously so that the muscles work against each other isometrically. In both cases we can also squeeze and flex the butt muscles at the same time—this creates synergy as the muscles pull together and push apart while contracting.

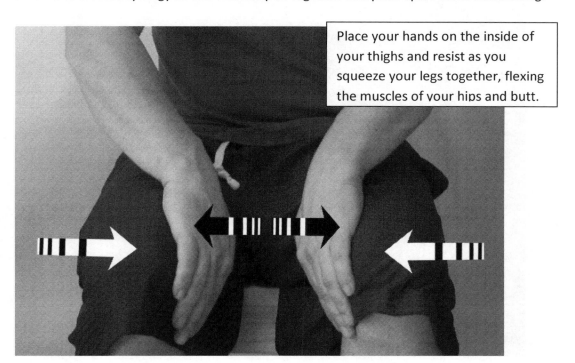

Place your hands on the inside of your thighs and resist as you squeeze your legs together, flexing the muscles of your hips and butt.

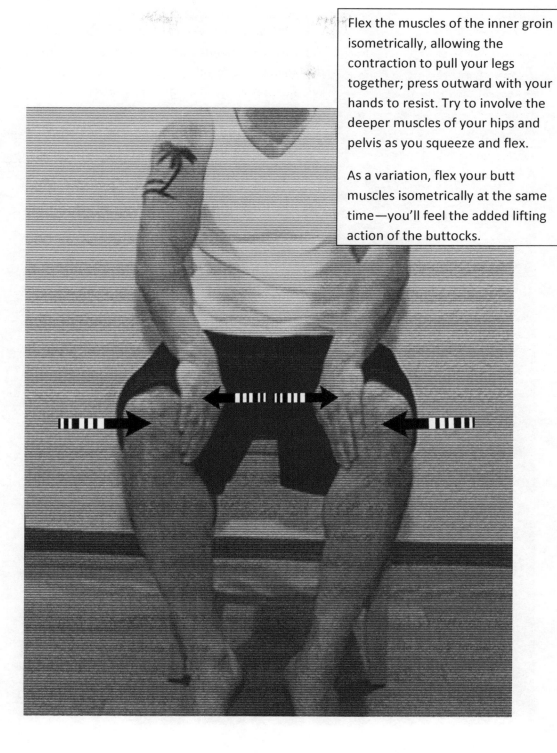

Flex the muscles of the inner groin isometrically, allowing the contraction to pull your legs together; press outward with your hands to resist. Try to involve the deeper muscles of your hips and pelvis as you squeeze and flex.

As a variation, flex your butt muscles isometrically at the same time—you'll feel the added lifting action of the buttocks.

With your knees closer together, the focus is on resisting the outward push of the hands, rather than squeezing the knees together. Activate and flex the pelvic floor, and try starting with your knees completely together. With your knees together and your femurs angled inward, you can feel the muscles in the sacral area flexing also.

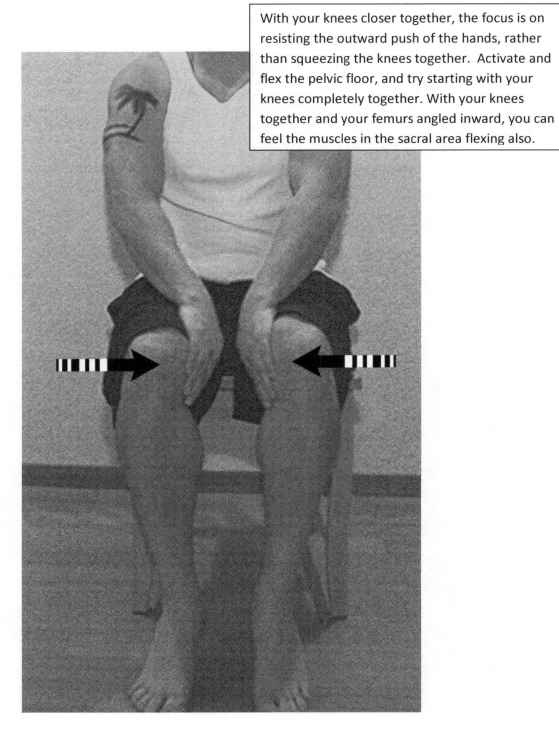

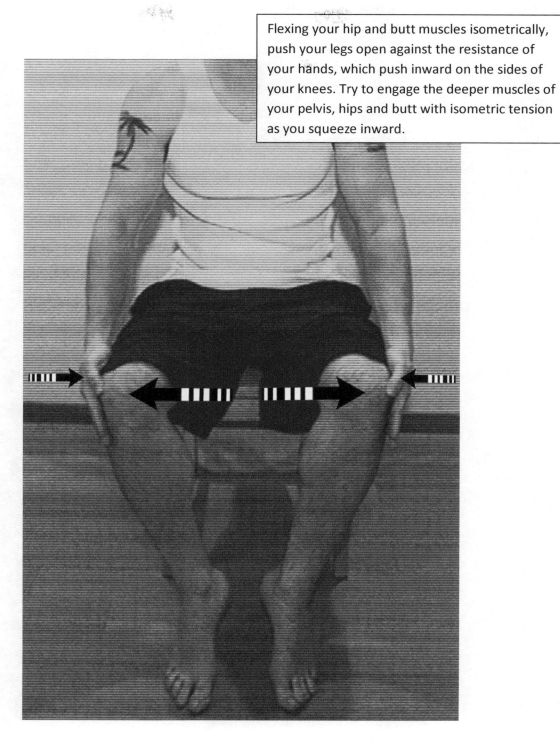

Flexing your hip and butt muscles isometrically, push your legs open against the resistance of your hands, which push inward on the sides of your knees. Try to engage the deeper muscles of your pelvis, hips and butt with isometric tension as you squeeze inward.

When your knees are wider apart than your hips, your femur bones point outward, forming a "V" shape from your pelvis. Pushing your legs *outward* from this position with isometric tension *increases* the flex of the butt muscles. Particularly if your feet are close together, your thighbones will tend to *rotate* outward, pulling your butt up and underneath you as it flexes. You can also try squeezing the butt muscles and the outer hips from this position *without* resistance from the hands.

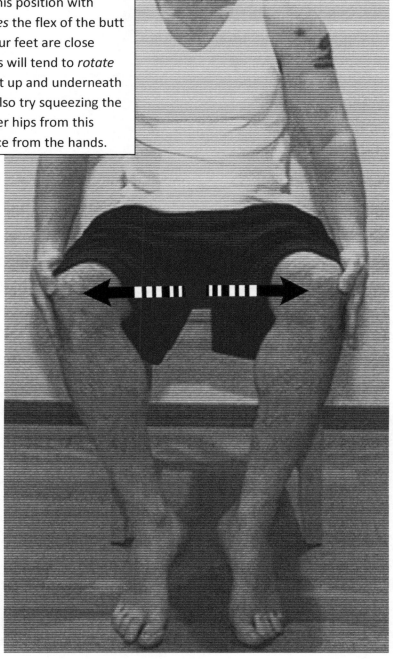

Isometric Core

What is the Core?

The Core is the functional center of your body—your muscular center-mass, consisting of the diaphragm, the abdominal muscles, the lower back and the pelvic floor. You can visualize your Core as a cylinder of muscle: the diaphragm is the top of the cylinder, the abdominal and lower back muscles are the sides, and the muscles of the pelvic floor are the bottom of the cylinder. The component muscles of the Core connect and interact in many complex ways; functionally, however, think of the Core as a cylinder of muscle extending from your diaphragm to your pelvic floor. The muscles of the Core are crucial to a healthy physique. The diaphragm powers the action of your breathing; the muscles of the pelvic floor support the intestines and the vital organs, and regulate the excretory and sexual functions; the abdominal and back muscles hold the body together and upright. Taken together, the Core is literally the center of strength in your body-- good posture, agility, coordination, power and fitness is ultimately rooted in your Core.

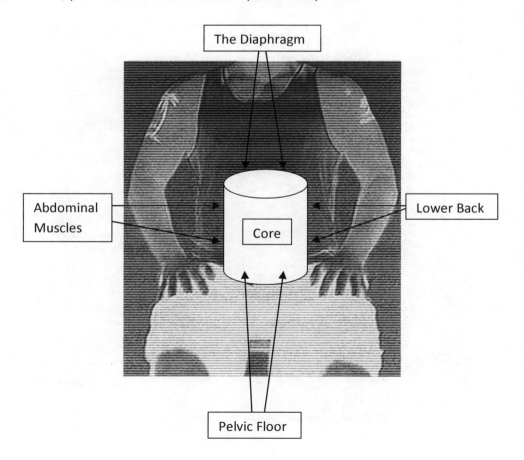

The Diaphragm

The diaphragm forms the top of the Core cylinder. It's a layer of muscle separating the upper and lower torso, which connects to the bottom of the rib cage and forms a convex seal between the lungs and heart above, and the viscera below.

When you inhale, the top of your diaphragm pulls downward, becoming concave. This *downward* pull of the diaphragm opens the rib cage and draws air into the lungs. Exhalation is the opposite: when you exhale, the top of the diaphragm pushes *upward* into a convex shape, pulling the ribs together and pushing air *from* the lungs.

Visualize the diaphragm *pulling downward* during inhalation, and *pushing upward* during exhalation from the *center* of your body.

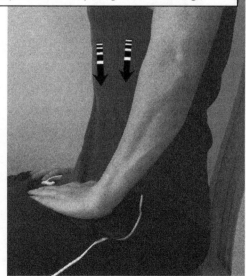

The diaphragm pushes *downward*, and the ribs expand *outward*, pulling air into the lungs.

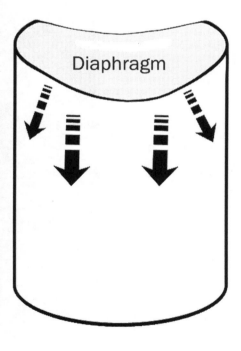

Inhalation

Diaphragm

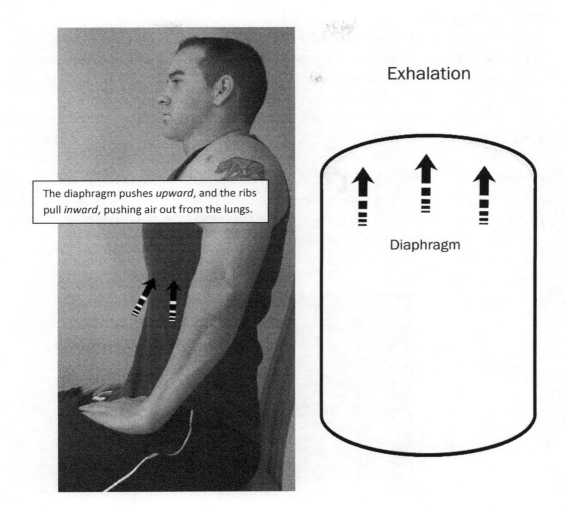

Exhalation

The diaphragm pushes *upward*, and the ribs pull *inward*, pushing air out from the lungs.

Diaphragm

This may seem counterintuitive at first, but as you become increasingly aware of the diaphragm *pulling downward* as you breathe in, and *pushing upward* as you breathe out, you'll get a deeper sense of both your breathing and your Core. Correct breathing technique revolves around this engagement of the diaphragm and the dynamic expansion and contraction of the rib cage. Breathing actively with the diaphragm will add energy and aliveness to everything you do, filling the lungs completely—front, side and rear—while activating and engaging the Core.

The Pelvic Floor

The pelvic floor is the bottom of the Core cylinder, just as the diaphragm is the top. The pelvic floor is the web of muscles that extend from the front of the pelvis to the spine, and includes the perineum and various other pelvic and lower abdominal muscles, which support the internal organs and are closely connected with the sexual and excretory systems. The PC muscle, which extends from the pubis to the tailbone, allows one to control urination and contracts involuntarily in cycles during sexual orgasm. Strengthening the PC muscle improves the health and fitness of the urinary tract and the reproductive system; it strengthens control over urination and ejaculation, and increases female orgasmic potential and vaginal tone; it is also very beneficial for the male prostate gland. Isometrically engaging your pelvic floor strengthens the bottom of your Core cylinder, synergistically increasing your total-body strength as well as your overall health.

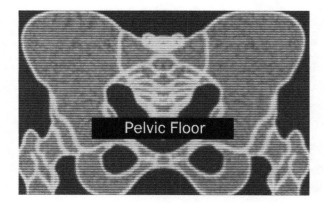

Pelvic Floor

Engaging the pelvic floor

When contracting the muscles of the pelvic floor, visualize them *pulling together* and *upwards*. Learn to contract the PC muscle in the same way that you would halt the flow of urine if you needed to stop peeing suddenly. Contract the muscles of the anus by squeezing in and lifting the anal mouth. These two contractions, together or separately, will tend to activate and flex the perineum area also; however keep in mind that it is possible to isolate the perineum and the inner pelvic muscles specifically using isometrics. Try to feel how all these muscles interconnect within your pelvis, and how they relate to the other muscles of the Core. Get a feel for how they respond to changes in your posture and breathing. As you become more adept, you will be able to control and differentiate the muscles in your lower regions more effectively; since the pelvic floor is the *base* of the Core, mastering pelvic muscle control will increase your overall Core strength and allow you to engage the *entire* Core more readily when practicing isometrics.

Kegel Exercises

The "Kegel" exercise, invented by Dr. Arnold Kegel, is the primary method to strengthen the PC muscle. To do the basic Kegel exercise contract your PC muscle as described above with moderate (60% - 80%) intensity and hold the contraction for approximately five seconds before releasing it. Rest a moment, and then repeat the contraction. Try doing 10 or 20 repetitions of this. Some experts recommend working up to 50 or 75 repetitions in a set, and repeating this 3-5 times a day; however I don't think you need to constrain yourself to a specific counting structure or number of repetitions in a day. If you do more on one day and less on another day, or a lot one week and absolutely none the next week, it really doesn't matter and you are still learning and progressing. As always, listen to your body.

Kegel variations

These are some variations for implementing the Kegel exercise. Remember to breathe.

1. Basic Kegel: Contract the PC muscle with moderate intensity and hold it for approximately 5 seconds, then release for approximately 2 or 3 seconds. Do between 10 and 100 repetitions in a set. Several sets a day is probably optimal.

2. The Kegel PC Flutter: In this variation, you contract the PC muscle very rapidly for a minimum of a few seconds (for beginners) up to about 1 minute for more advanced practitioners. You will probably find that "fluttering" or rapidly contracting the PC in this manner seems tricky at first and the PC muscle quickly becomes fatigued; work at it and you will quickly get stronger and more coordinated, and should be able to do 30 second or 1-minute flutter sequences easily.

3. The Kegel extended hold: Flex the PC muscle and hold the contraction. Aim for a moderately intense contraction, and see if you can hold it for 1 minute or so and then rest. In the beginning, you may find that holding a 1-minute Kegel contraction can be challenging, however don't get discouraged. With practice and concentration you'll easily be able hold a contraction for a minute or more.

Remember to breathe naturally and to not overstrain or over-flex your PC; and be sure to let your PC muscle really RELAX after working it. Release your grip, breathe into the perineum area, and release any residual tension. As with all our isometric training, learning to use isometrics and to flex a muscle group effectively also entails learning how to RELAX that muscle group as well. Kegels are no different, and learning to relax the PC and other deep muscles of the pelvis will add real value to your practice.

Yoga and the pelvic floor

In yoga, the practice of flexing and strengthening the perineum and the pelvic floor muscles extends into the practice of what's known as bandhas, or locks, and pranayama, or breath control.

Horse mudra

In yoga, the concentrated contraction of the anal sphincter muscles is called Horse Mudra. In practice Horse Mudra would usually be combined with some type of breath control or pranayama—one example would be contracting the anus and the entire anal mouth upward as you inhale, and then holding that inhalation and the contraction for a few seconds, then releasing the anus and exhaling. According to Yoga theory, this contraction or "locking" of the anus while holding the in-breath, generates and pulls energy upward in the body, especially through spine. This type of technique is considered to be invigorating and rejuvenating for the nervous system.

An advanced insight here is that inhalation in general corresponds to the tensing of the smooth muscles of the digestive and circulatory systems. You may realize that when defecating there is an instinct sometimes to inhale and hold your breath as if building up pressure to expel a bowel movement—inhaling and holding the breath is actually causing the colon to contract involuntarily. Similarly, the veins and arteries of the circulatory system subtly contract and relax with the inhalation and exhalation of the breath; this concept is useful for maintaining steady blood pressure while using isometrics, and can be a useful tool for releasing tightness and tension trapped in the body.

Mula bandha

In yoga, Mula bandha, or the "root lock", is the contraction of the center of the perineum. The spot midway between the anus and the sex organs, and approximately one inch inside the body, is subtly contracted without involving or contracting the anal or PC muscles. In Yoga practice, one would contract this point while inhaling, and hold the contraction for a few seconds with the in-breath, and then exhale and release the contraction. In Yoga theory, this spot, roughly, is known as the Muladhara Chakra, one of the primary subtle energy centers of the body; Mula Bandha, the root lock, is thought to energize the body and mind and to pull energy *upwards* into the spine. I mention Mula Bandha here to present an additional and slightly more subtle perspective on the PC and pelvic floor muscles. Keep in mind that there is always another level to these techniques beyond the merely mechanical. Experiment, listen to your body, and see what you can learn, discover and figure out.

Full isometric Core contraction

When we work the Core with isometrics, we flex the lower back and ab muscles, breathe actively with the diaphragm and lift the pelvic floor—squeezing the Core cylinder from all sides at once. When working with the Core, think about the concept of muscular counter-tension: when you breathe in your ribs *expand*, but while your ribs expand outward, your abdominal muscles are squeezing *inward*, and your lower back muscles are extending your spine *upward*. So in a sense you're pulling with your core muscles in several different directions at once; this kind of counter-tension allows you to hold yourself upright in space, and also to intensely work your Core using isometrics. Work with the concept of the Core as a cylinder. Pull the Core together from top to bottom by lifting the pelvic floor and pushing downward with the diaphragm; squeeze it from the sides by flexing the abdominal and back muscles, and extend and lengthen your spine upward. Balance the counter-tensions of the Core muscles against each other with muscle control, and flex your Core isometrically.

Core contraction techniques

Note that while only technique #5 and technique #6 are specifically suited for use at the poker table, all of these techniques are useful to develop, strengthen and get in touch with your Core.

Technique #1: Lie down on your back with your feet placed flat on the ground and your knees bent. Exhale, and gently but firmly pull your belly button downward toward your spine. Allow your abdomen to flatten or "hollow" if possible. [Tip: It sometimes helps to "let go" and allow gravity to pull your belly button down as you exhale, *then* pull inward.]

Technique #2: Lie down on your back with your feet placed flat on the ground and your knees bent. Contract your PC and pelvic floor muscles. Now exhale, and pull your belly button toward your spine, as in technique #1.

Technique #3: Stand with your hands on your hips, placing your thumbs on your abdomen just above the pelvis. Imagine that you are cinching a belt tightly around your waist, contracting and pulling in the muscles of your abdomen and lower back. Continue to breathe actively with your diaphragm, opening your rib cage while inhaling.

Technique #4: Stand with your hands on your hips, placing your thumbs on your abdomen just above the pelvis. Contract your PC and your pelvic floor lifting it upwards. Now imagine that you are cinching a belt tightly around your waist, contracting and pulling in the muscles of your abdomen and lower back.

Technique #5: From a lying, standing or sitting position contract the pelvic floor; contract the muscles of the lower back, extending your spine upwards; and contract and squeeze your abdominal muscles, pulling the belly button toward the spine.

Technique #6: From a lying, standing or sitting position squeeze the abdomen inward from the front and sides, and contract the pelvic floor muscles, lifting the pelvic floor upward. Breathe actively into your ribs, feeling the diaphragm's downward push as you inhale, and the pulling together of the ribs as you exhale.

As you practice and experiment with these techniques, and discover new ones, remember the principle of muscular counter-tension. Feel how various muscles support and resist each other, and the ways they pull apart, or toward, each other. Look for isometric sweet spots, where the tension in the Core feels lively and dynamic. Keep in mind that what we are calling the Core is also regarded as central by Yoga and all the martial arts. Your Core is the center of your physical being, the center of physical movement and is your center of your balance.

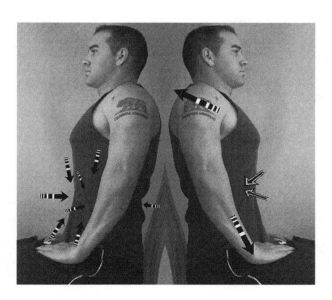

Strengthening the isometric Core at the poker table

When we use isometrics to strengthen the Core at the poker table we must be careful not to strain or hold our breath, so that we don't excessively elevate our blood pressure.

> **CAUTION: DO NOT OVER-SQUEEZE YOUR ABDOMEN, STRAIN, OR HOLD YOUR BREATH WHEN USING ISOMETRICS ON YOUR CORE IN A SITTING POSITION. When working with the Core, use only moderate isometric tension for brief intervals, keep your neck and face relaxed, and breathe normally. If you feel dizzy, lightheaded, or short of breath for any reason, stop immediately.**

When you use isometrics on your Core while playing poker, you first of all want to be discrete—you certainly don't want to appear like you're physically straining or doing some kind of abdominal crunches at the table. You also don't want to elevate or spike your blood pressure, so be sure to keep breathing during isometric contractions, and not overstrain.

All of the positions and techniques in this chapter are to be combined with a *moderate* full Core contraction as we have already described. You may find that with some practice, merely breathing into the ribcage with your diaphragm will give you the feeling of your Core starting to engage. When you add to that a contraction and lifting of the pelvic floor, now the bottom *and* the top of your Core are getting involved. If you then sit up straight, extending your spine upward, and pull your navel inward toward your spine, gently flexing your abdominal and lower back muscles—now you are doing full isometric Core contraction. Be aware that you can shift the focus and intensity of the isometric contraction into specific areas: while keeping your Core flexed and activated, you can for instance contract one side or the other more strongly, or pull one muscle away from another. With practice, you'll find that merely sitting up straight in your chair as you lightly flex your Core and twisting imperceptibly to one side can have a tremendous strengthening effect on your abs and obliques. The key is the way you actively engage the muscles isometrically and balance their force against each other. Just gaining this awareness will literally tighten up your abs.

Remember, all these techniques are done from stationary positions—you're not moving your body around. Good technique is to engage your Core and then to shift into position for a specific technique and just hold it there, continuing to work your Core contraction and breathing normally. All of the adjustments and actions described are taking place *internally*, as your work with isometrics against your own muscular counter-tension. Even a close observer should not be able to notice what you're doing.

Push downward with your hands onto your thighs as you flex your ab muscles and activate your Core. As the contraction of your abs pulls you forward, you resist by lifting upward with your back muscles and your arms; this is a *stationary* position. Breathe normally and don't overstrain. A moderate contraction and isometric activation of the Core is what we are aiming for.

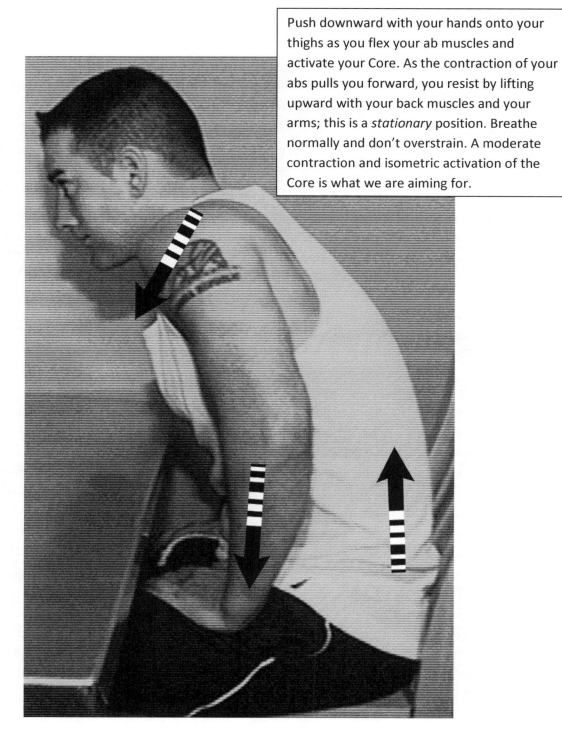

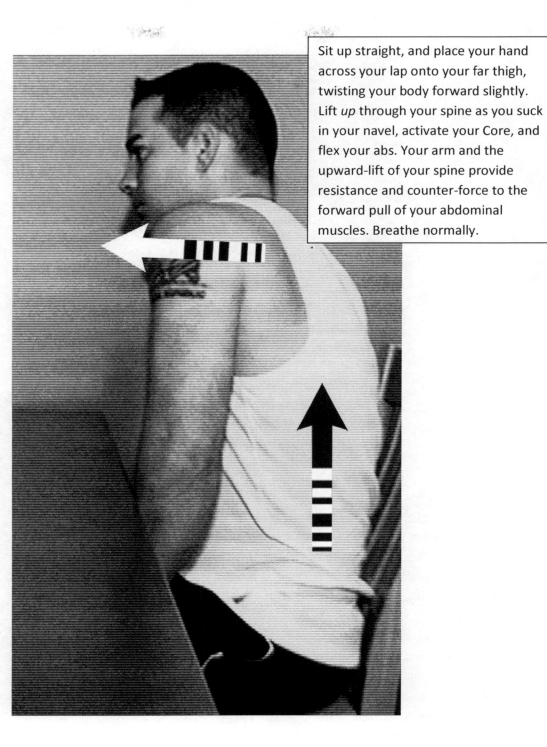

Sit up straight, and place your hand across your lap onto your far thigh, twisting your body forward slightly. Lift *up* through your spine as you suck in your navel, activate your Core, and flex your abs. Your arm and the upward-lift of your spine provide resistance and counter-force to the forward pull of your abdominal muscles. Breathe normally.

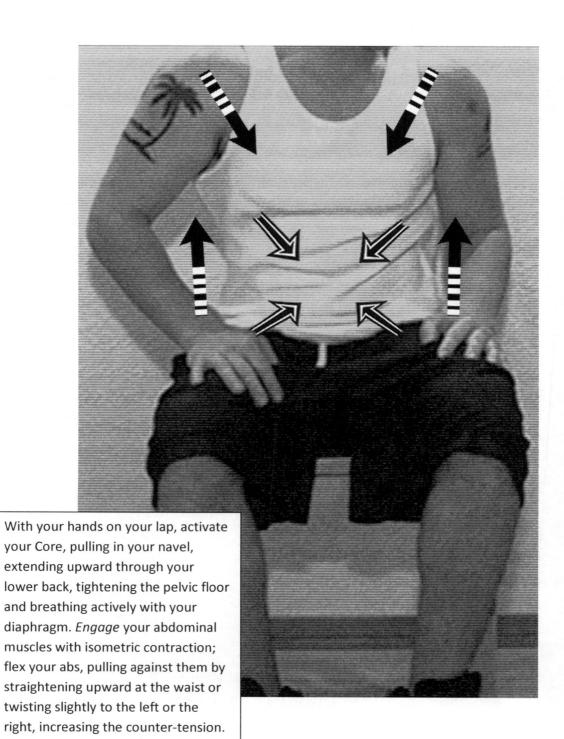

With your hands on your lap, activate your Core, pulling in your navel, extending upward through your lower back, tightening the pelvic floor and breathing actively with your diaphragm. *Engage* your abdominal muscles with isometric contraction; flex your abs, pulling against them by straightening upward at the waist or twisting slightly to the left or the right, increasing the counter-tension.

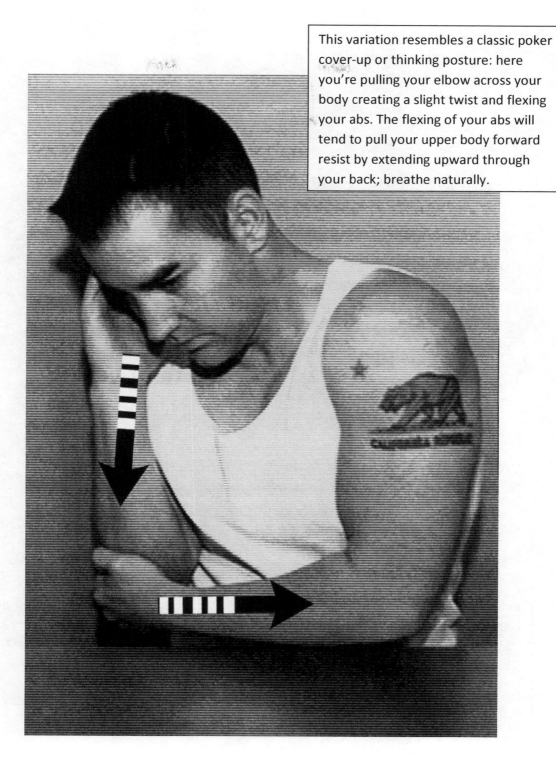

This variation resembles a classic poker cover-up or thinking posture: here you're pulling your elbow across your body creating a slight twist and flexing your abs. The flexing of your abs will tend to pull your upper body forward resist by extending upward through your back; breathe naturally.

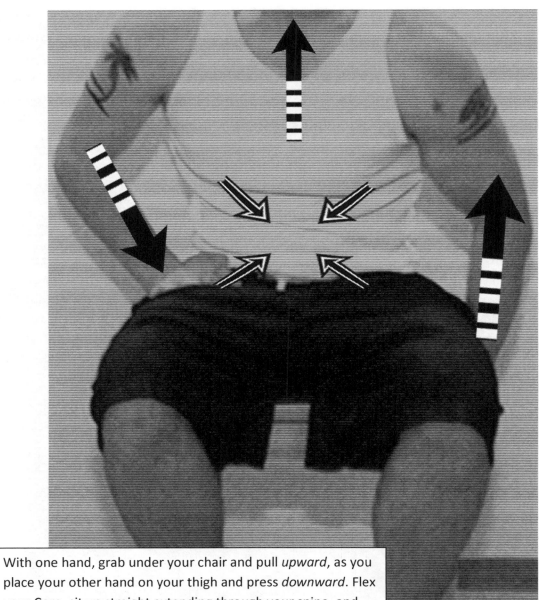

With one hand, grab under your chair and pull *upward*, as you place your other hand on your thigh and press *downward*. Flex your Core, sit up straight extending through your spine, and let the isometric contraction of your abs stabilize your body, as you simultaneously lift yourself upward and pull yourself downward. Remember to breathe normally and to keep your head and face relaxed; don't strain.

Isometric Hands and Forearms

The forearms are a great target for isometric training, especially when playing poker; and getting an isometric pump in your forearm muscles feels great and is a true stress reliever; it can also increase mental alertness, strengthen your grip and reduce your risk of arthritis and carpal tunnel syndrome. Although our hands and forearms are extremely complex, and our wrists and fingers can move in an infinite variety of ways, when working with isometrics we can focus on the large muscles on the top and bottom of the forearm, and the tendons and muscles of the wrist, hands and fingers.

> CAUTION: If you've been diagnosed with Carpal Tunnel syndrome or Arthritis, or suffer from persistent pain in your hands or wrists, you should consult a physician before doing any of the exercises in this section.

The primary method to flex the hands and forearms is also the most obvious: make a tight fist. If you squeeze your fist tightly, you will flex the muscles of your hands and fingers, as well as those of your wrist and forearm. This simple action can, if combined with proper isometric technique, effectively build strong hands and forearms very easily. Think of the flexed-fist as the foundation of isometric hand and forearm training. Focus on isolating the contraction in your hands and forearms, and avoid tensing your upper arms and shoulders. Breathe naturally, sustain the contraction, and focus on the muscles of each finger, as well as your palm, the back of your hand, and the tendons of your wrist.

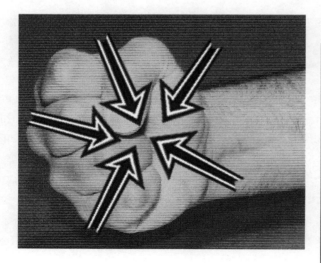

Roll your hand into a fist, fingers first. Escalate the tension in your grip into an intense *squeeze*, flexing your forearm. Breathe normally as you hold the contraction.

When you let go, allow your hand and forearm to fully relax and release any excess stored tension or stress.

Try curling your wrist toward you, as you squeeze your fist tightly. Focus on flexing the muscles on the underside of your forearm. As before, breathe naturally, ramp smoothly into a firm contraction, and hold it; relax your muscles when you let go. For added torque, straighten your elbow away from you as your curl your wrist toward you.

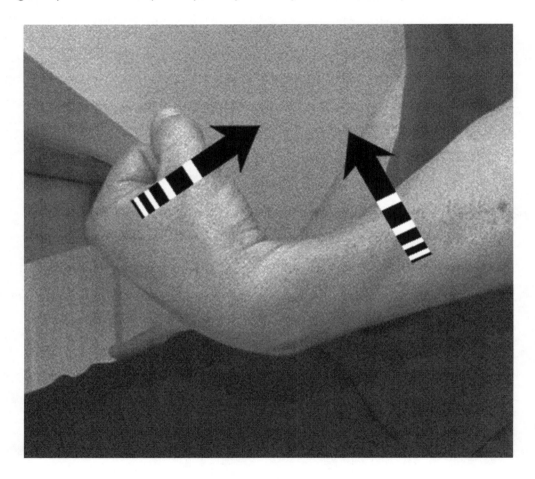

Spreading your fingers wide flexes and activates the tendons of your wrist—if you grab your wrist with your other hand you can feel your wrist flexing and expanding when you do this. This is the opposite of *squeezing* your fist—spread your fingers outward as far as you can, and hold this position for a few seconds, focusing on the extension and flex of the wrist tendons. Eventually you'll get more of a feel for which fingers flex which tendons, and how to extend your strength right through the tips of your fingers. Also, try spreading your fingers wide with your palm pressed into the table for a slightly different effect.

By forcefully spreading your fingers as wide as you can, you activate and flex the tendons of your wrist. Stretch your fingers wide apart, outward from the center of your hand. Notice the way your wrist widens and flexes as you do this.

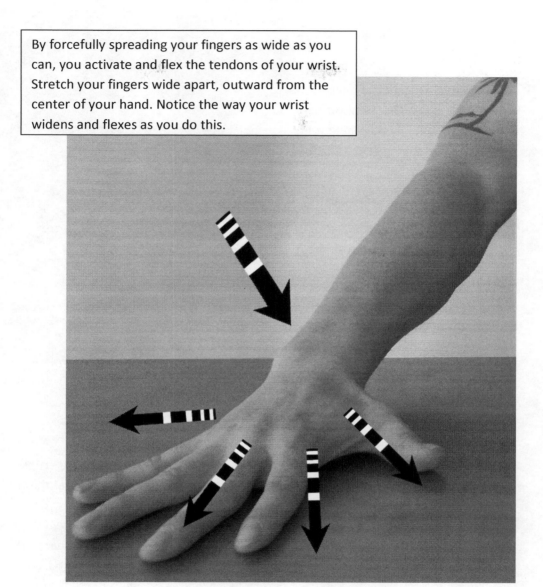

Next, we're going to focus on the fingers specifically. We can use isometrics to work the fingers by pressing them into the table and contracting the finger muscles, pulling the fingers together or spreading them slightly apart; bending them, and straightening them. Use moderate isometric tension on the fingers, and don't force them—try to engage the finger muscles with isometrics and the leverage of the table; you'll feel results quickly with even minimal effort.

Press down *gently* onto the table, protecting your cards. Squeeze your finger muscles as if pulling your fingers together right through the table. Feel how the tendons in your wrist flex and expand as you do this. Now try pulling just *one finger* at a time inward, and notice which tendon in your wrist flexes and pops out as you do so. Now, press downward and outward with your fingers as if spreading the table apart. Focus on the contraction of the muscles and tendons of your wrist and fingers.

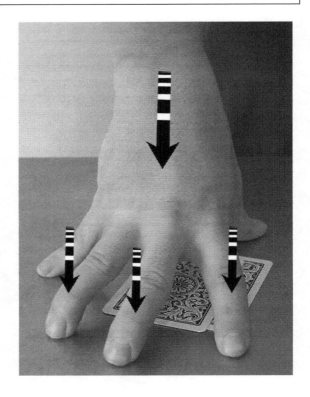

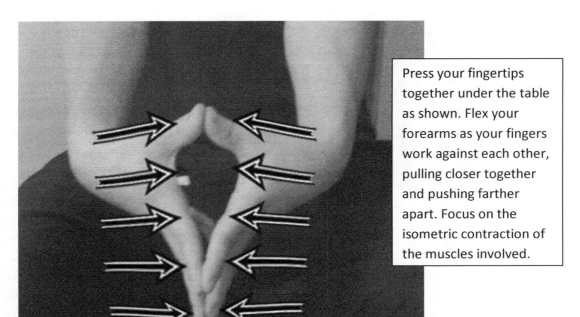

Press your fingertips together under the table as shown. Flex your forearms as your fingers work against each other, pulling closer together and pushing farther apart. Focus on the isometric contraction of the muscles involved.

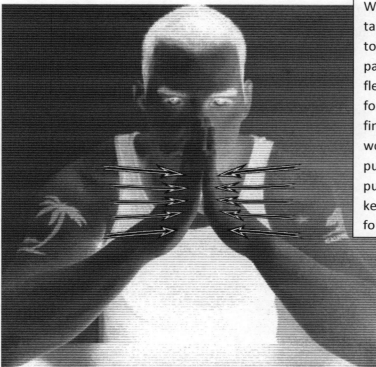

With your elbows on the table, touch your fingers together and press your palms toward each other, flexing your wrists and forearms. Keeping your fingers pressed together, work between the actions of pulling your palms apart and pushing them together, keeping the wrists and forearms flexed.

Pressing the fingertips together; notice that your palms don't touch: like two magnetic poles repelling each other, they press apart with isometric tension as your wrists bend forward, pushing your fingertips together.

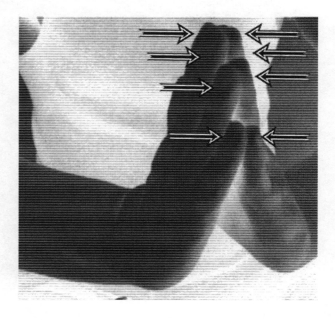

Now we'll work on bending the wrist backward or forward, applying resistance with the other hand. Keep in mind these techniques are to be done with only minimal movement if any—only very slight changes in angle or position. Flexing your wrist backward you'll feel the contraction mostly on the back of your wrist and your forearm; curling your wrist forward you'll feel it more on the front of your forearm. Mix and match the wrist angles and the direction of force and resistance: try pulling your wrist back further when it's already bent backward, and also try pulling it forward from that position; with your wrist bent forward, try pulling it further forward, or flexing it backward; and with a straight wrist try flexing the wrist back or forward, always resisting with the opposite hand. Also try letting the opposite hand actively pull or push the wrist—and then use isometric tension to flex your wrist and forearm as you resist.

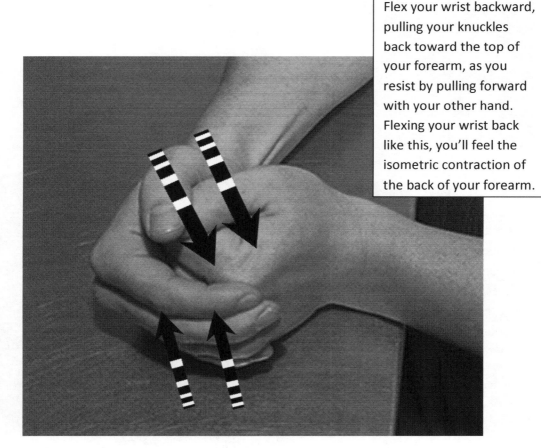

Flex your wrist backward, pulling your knuckles back toward the top of your forearm, as you resist by pulling forward with your other hand. Flexing your wrist back like this, you'll feel the isometric contraction of the back of your forearm.

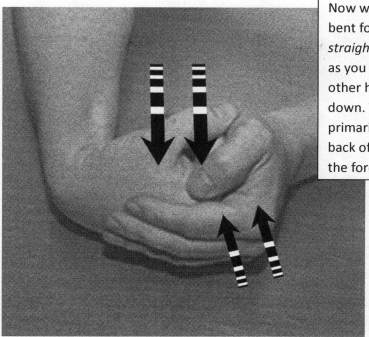

Now with your wrist bent forward, work to *straighten* your wrist, as you resist with your other hand, holding it down. This is again primarily working the back of the wrist and the forearm.

Starting again with your wrist bent backward, now push your wrist *forward*, as you resist with the top hand. You are curling your wrist toward the straight position here, primarily flexing the underside of your forearm.

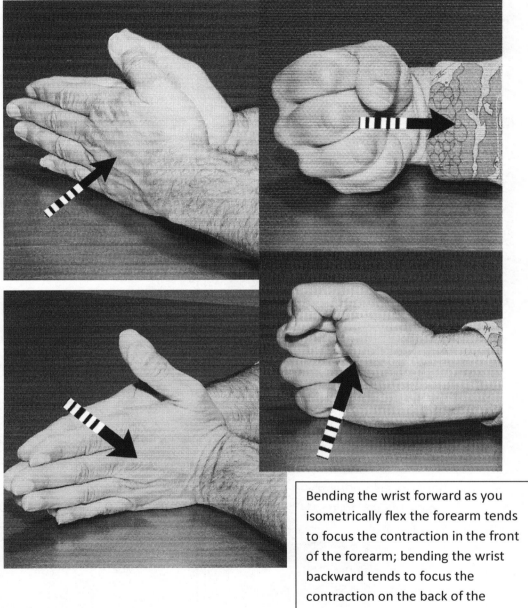

Bending the wrist forward as you isometrically flex the forearm tends to focus the contraction in the front of the forearm; bending the wrist backward tends to focus the contraction on the back of the forearm.

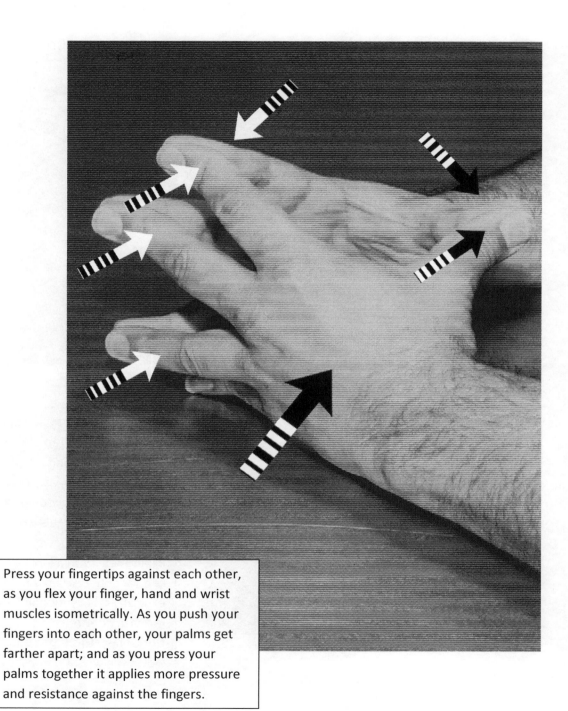

Press your fingertips against each other, as you flex your finger, hand and wrist muscles isometrically. As you push your fingers into each other, your palms get farther apart; and as you press your palms together it applies more pressure and resistance against the fingers.

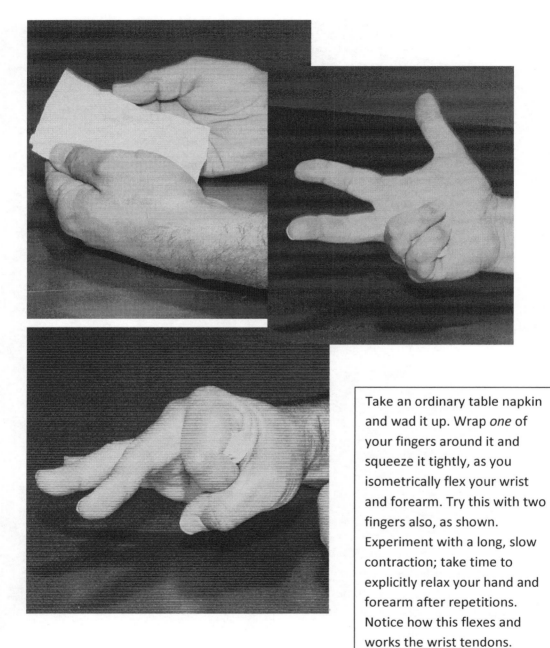

Take an ordinary table napkin and wad it up. Wrap *one* of your fingers around it and squeeze it tightly, as you isometrically flex your wrist and forearm. Try this with two fingers also, as shown. Experiment with a long, slow contraction; take time to explicitly relax your hand and forearm after repetitions. Notice how this flexes and works the wrist tendons.

Isometrics at the gym

Many poker players do manage to get to the gym occasionally, which is of course a good thing. When you train with weights or resistance machines, you'll find that you can incorporate isometric techniques and concepts very readily. With the increased focus and muscle control that you've gained from doing isometrics, you'll be able to maximize the value of lifting weights or working on machines—a few simple reps on a triceps machine, for example, when combined with isometric tension at key spots in your range of motion, can become an exquisitely intense arm workout. Since you've become proficient at flexing your muscles with nothing but internal resistance using isometrics, and focusing on the *quality* of the muscular contraction, you'll *really* ramp things up when you hit the gym: a gym full of weights and resistance machines will start to look more like a playground to you. And none of this requires lifting heavy weights either—just enough resistance to effectively engage your muscles is all you really need.

An isometric muscular contraction does not shorten the muscles involved or move the body; but when you're lifting weights or working with resistance machines your muscles will be engaged in *isotonic* contraction—they'll be shortening as they contract and your body will be moving through a range of motion as you do repetitions. We incorporate isometrics into resistance training by adding in isometric contraction: stopping at key points in a repetition and flexing the muscles isometrically, and then smoothly blending that isometric contraction back into an isotonic one and continuing the exercise. At points of overload or failure, when we're stopped and can't move the weight any further, we take advantage of the opportunity to squeeze the muscle isometrically, which greatly increases the muscle's workload.

Guidelines for integrating isometrics with resistance weight training

1. Focus on the muscular contraction first—let your *muscles* move the weight.
2. The goal is intense, targeted muscular contractions, not moving weights around.
3. Look for points in your range of motion to slow down, stop and squeeze your muscles with isometric contraction.
4. Apply isometrics to muscles that are fully extended or stretched.
5. Apply isometrics to muscles that are fully shortened and contracted.
6. Utilize negative resistance by flexing your muscles with isometric force as they lengthen on the reverse of a repetition—for example, when you lower a weight bar.
7. The machines and weights are just tools for you to flex your muscles against; always keep your focus pointed inward onto what your muscles are doing.

Opening your back

Floor back opening #1

One of the first things I emphasize in Yoga, even before Downward Dog, is the concept of letting go of back-tension. Lying flat on your stomach is a great way to start: as you lie face-down on a flat surface, the stress of standing, sitting and walking is removed from your spine, and the force of gravity and your own body weight gently pulls your spine downward, restoring its natural curve. Bring your focus into your back, and try to feel where you're storing tension or soreness. When you find tension, make an effort to let it go, to release it.

The concept of "breathing into" tense or sore areas relates tangentially to what we've said about the relation of inhalation and exhalation to the involuntary smooth muscles such as blood vessels. *Inhalation* corresponds with contraction, while *exhalation* corresponds to relaxation; breathing into an area of stored tension in the body allows us to voluntarily tense it and thus to take control of that tension, and then to consciously release it as we exhale. This is also happening on a vascular level as well, as the blood vessels will contract slightly on the inhalation, and dilate slightly on the exhalation; and when we relax a tense area of our body we are allowing for greater circulation to that area. If you observe yourself carefully, you'll notice that when, for instance, you're working on a difficult math problem you may inhale sharply and hold your breath as you concentrate—this can at times be an unconscious way of forcing blood into a particular area of the brain, or of attempting to hold concentration on single point. Of course, the exact opposite of this can just as well be true, and people can vary greatly in their abilities and tendencies. I only bring this idea up to draw attention to the role of the inhalation and exhalation in affecting the vascular system.

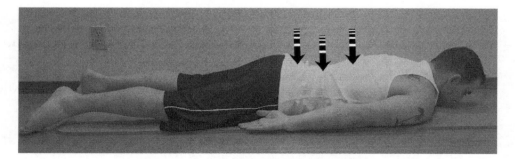

Breathe *into* any tense or sore area of your back; as you inhale, feel the area gently tighten; as you exhale, let go of all the tension in that area, as you relax all your spinal nerves and muscles. Allow your back to *lengthen* with the pull of gravity; allow your vertebrae to spread, and your back to open.

Floor back opening #2

Now lie on your back with your knees bent and your feet flat on the floor. Relax your back and neck; breathe actively into your ribs, letting your diaphragm open the rib cage from the center of your body. Push with your hands against your thighs, lengthening your spine and pushing your shoulders away from your hips. Combine this natural traction with a focus on your breathing: opening your rib cage and filling the lungs in all directions as you push downward against your thighs and extend your spine, pulling it upward from the pelvis.

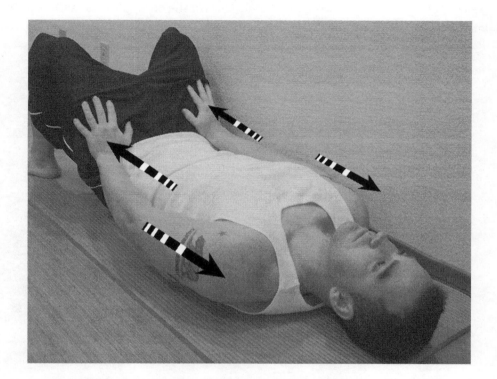

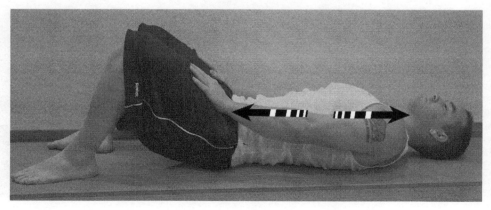

Floor back opening #3

Now, lift your hips upward toward the ceiling. Keeping your shoulders flat, press your feet downward into the floor and push your pelvis upward. Hold this position for a few seconds at a time. When practicing this technique start with a deep inhalation, then pull your tailbone under, and push it upward through your hips toward the ceiling. Exaggerate the curve of your back, arching upward and bridging onto your shoulders; as you arch focus on opening the *front* of your spine. The primary action here is the triangle of the tailbone pushing directly upward through the body toward the ceiling; as you arch your back breathe into the front of your spine, and open your chest.

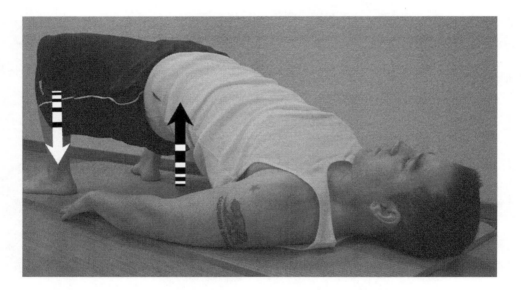

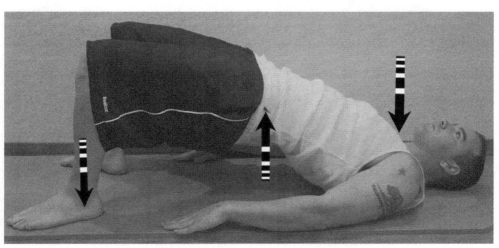

Standing back opening #1

The following position is one of the very best back openers. The central concept with this position is the relationship between the stretch of the hamstring muscles and the extension and lengthening of the spine. Place your elbows on the tops of your thighs and bend your legs comfortably. Allow your back to flatten out and lengthen. Do not hunch your back. Stick your butt out in an exaggerated manner, relax, bend your knees deeply, put your weight back onto your legs and your elbows, and extend your back so it's flat, like a table, creating a straight line between your hips and the back of your head. Release tension from the back.

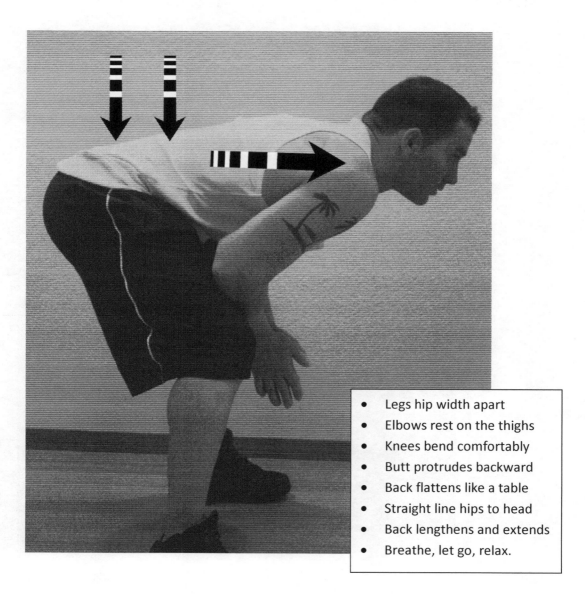

- Legs hip width apart
- Elbows rest on the thighs
- Knees bend comfortably
- Butt protrudes backward
- Back flattens like a table
- Straight line hips to head
- Back lengthens and extends
- Breathe, let go, relax.

Now, keeping your elbows on your thighs and maintaining a flat back, straighten your knees up. You'll notice immediately that this creates a stretching action in your hamstring muscles, and the tendency will be for your back to pull tighter and curve or hunch in compensation. Resist this, and work to keep your back flat and your spine extending outwards toward your head. You can imagine that this position is the same as if you were seated and touching your toes—the straighter your back, the more it pulls on your hamstrings. Keep the back straight and don't overstretch.

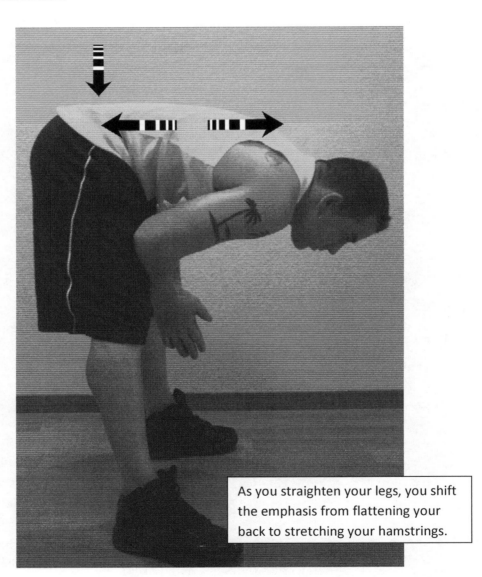

As you straighten your legs, you shift the emphasis from flattening your back to stretching your hamstrings.

Now bend your knees again, sticking your butt out and placing your weight onto your elbows; sink *into* your legs, knees and elbows, releasing and extending your back. Take your time and rest here. This is an extremely restorative position; it takes all the pressure off your back and allows you to extend and relax your spine. Breathe into your back and focus on relaxing the spinal muscles and allowing the vertebrae and disks to decompress. This is a very good restorative stretch to practice in the shower, also, provided you have a safe shower with non-slip mats: let the hot water pour down on your lower back and massage it as you release the tension from your back, extend your spine, and relax.

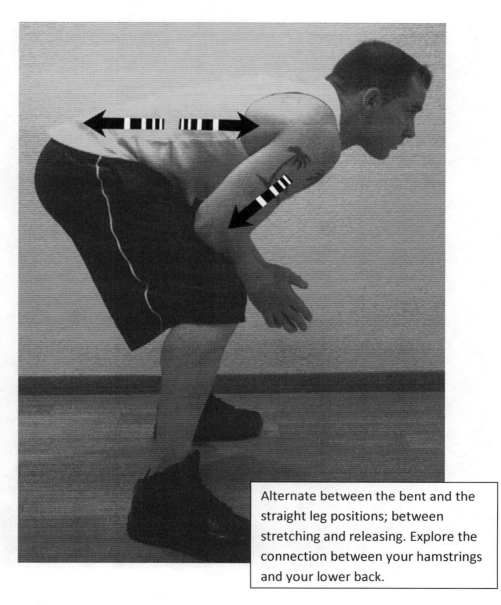

Alternate between the bent and the straight leg positions; between stretching and releasing. Explore the connection between your hamstrings and your lower back.

Standing back opening #2

With your legs straight and hip width apart reach toward the ground, allowing yourself to release forward and downward, your arms hanging to the floor. Let the weight of your upper body descend between your legs, and release your lower back. Keep your legs active and engaged by pressing your feet into the floor, flexing your quads and lifting your kneecaps upward as you stretch forward with your legs straight. Try to *let go* with your back and let your upper body hang downward, your spine lengthening and your rib cage moving away from your hips.

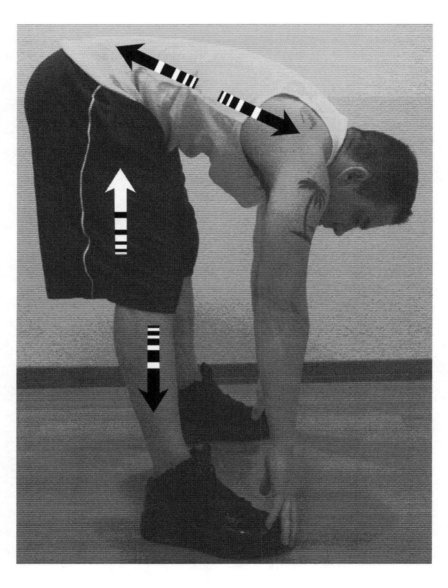

As you come out of the forward stretch, place your elbows on your knees, let your weight sink back into your haunches, extend your spine forward and flatten your back. Relax for a moment, allowing your back to align itself before you straighten up into a standing posture.

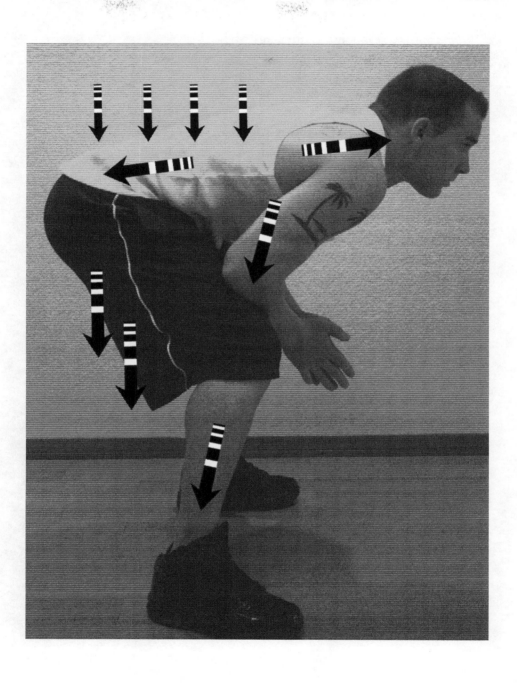

Standing back opening #3

Stand with your feet hip-width apart and interlock your fingers, pressing your palms upward toward the ceiling.

As you press your hands upward, extend your body and lengthen your spine. Feel your spine lengthening and pulling *upward* from within your pelvis.

Keep your legs solidly planted on the floor, and as you press upward feel the stretch, as if your hands were being pulled toward the ceiling and your feet were being pulled downward. Maintain an *active Core* as you extend, breathing into your ribs with your diaphragm and filling up the front, sides and back of your lungs with fresh air.

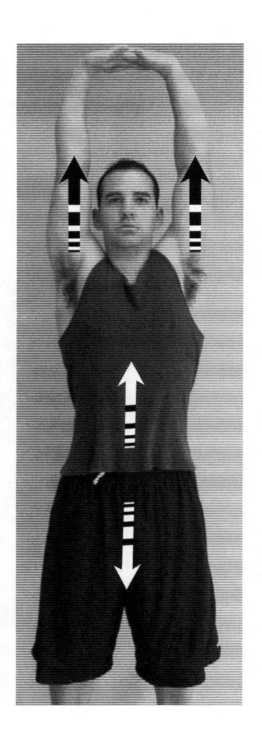

Now, lean over to the side about 20 or 30 degrees. Continue pressing upward with your palms and extending your spine up from your pelvis. As you lean to one side, feel the other side of your spine stretch and open.

Come back to center and stretch upwards again, and then lean to the opposite side and again press upwards and outwards with your palms. Focus on the action of the spine as it bends sideways; *feel* it stretching and opening.

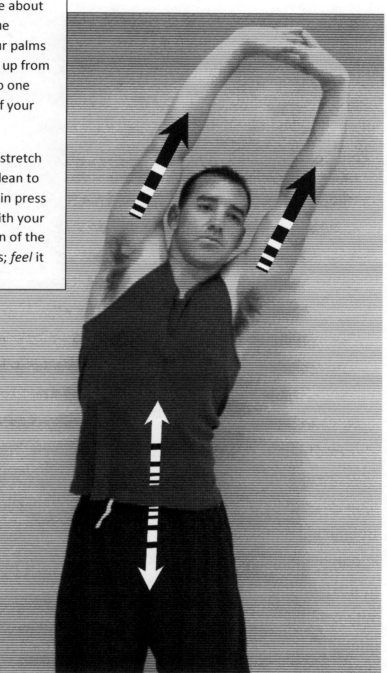

Standing back opening #4

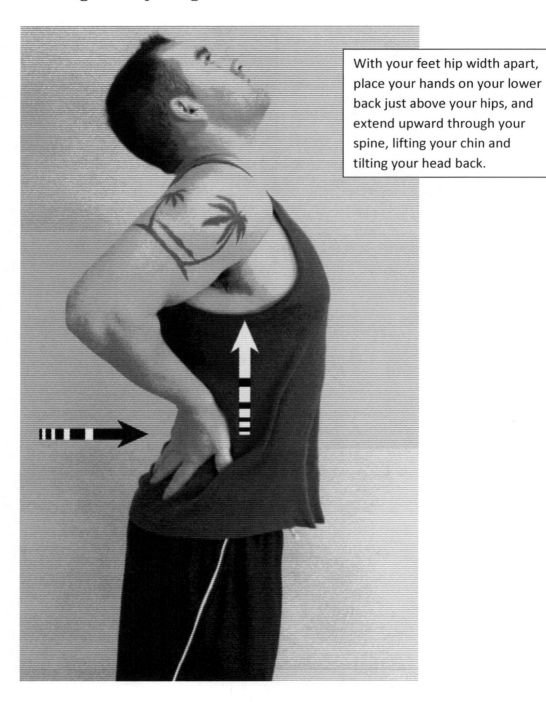

With your feet hip width apart, place your hands on your lower back just above your hips, and extend upward through your spine, lifting your chin and tilting your head back.

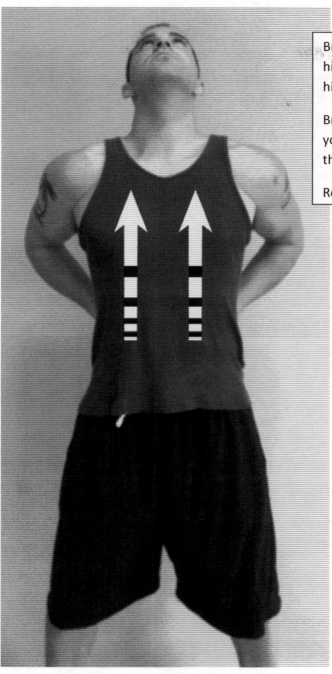

Bracing your hands against your hips, arch backward, pushing your hips forward.

Breathe into your lower back as you arch, and focus on opening the *front* of your spine.

Return to a standing position.

Poker nutrition

Eating healthy and losing weight

What a person eats is a very personal subject and I'm not about to say that what anybody eats is necessarily right or wrong. Humans, like bears, are omnivorous; and while some people eat lots of pasta or noodles every day, others eat nothing but meat and vegetables; some people eat nothing but rice and tofu, while others eat nothing but fast food. At the furthest extremes, some people eat almost nothing but protein shakes and vitamins, while others consume nothing but coffee, candy and donuts. But between such extremes lie the vast numbers of personal diet variations—which for many of us are fairly random and can be different every day, depending on what we happen to be eating at the moment.

If you already know what you're doing regarding diet and nutrition, feel free to skim this chapter or to skip it altogether. However, if you feel like you could improve on your current diet, what follows is a simple dietary program for losing weight, increasing lean muscle mass, improving cardiovascular health, lowering bad cholesterol (LDL), increasing good cholesterol (HDL), improving hormonal balance and boosting your energy level. While anyone could argue that there are more optimally balanced and comprehensive diets out there, the system presented here is firmly grounded on well-known principles of nutrition, and is simplified and structured so that anybody, even a busy poker player who eats many meals in casinos and restaurants, can easily stick with it. There is no calorie counting, portion sizing or complexity; and this diet allows for the occasional cheat meal or cheat day, so you don't ever have to feel deprived.

The Simple Poker Diet

This diet, the Simple Poker Diet, focuses on eating lots of high quality lean protein and lots of delicious vegetables—foods which you can always find on a casino menu if you try. At the end of this section, there are some healthy casino meal recommendations: Chicken Satay with Sunomuno salad, for example, or broiled swordfish with mixed vegetables. We're not going to get into a complex discussion about nutritional science here; however this diet *is* based on nutritional principles well known to be conducive to muscular development, weight loss, higher testosterone levels (for men), better sleep, and a decreased risk of heart disease. This diet will also eliminate most heartburn, indigestion, constipation, headaches and joint pain.

GUIDELINES

- Eat between 2 to 6 reasonably sized meals a day, consisting of foods from **Group A.**
- There are no explicit restrictions on portion sizes or caloric intake; however, moderation is usually a good thing. You will probably find that if you follow the diet's guidelines you will suffer much less from food cravings, which are often exacerbated by eating foods high in simple carbohydrates, like bread or pastries.
- Balance your meals with different combinations of lean protein, vegetables and legumes: protein-legumes; vegetables-legumes; protein-vegetables; protein-vegetables-legumes, and so forth. This will improve your results and keep you satisfied, and your energy levels high.
- Feel free to take a day off from the diet once a week, or to have a cheat meal every few days. Many bodybuilders use a six-meals-on, one-meal-off approach, or a six-days-on, one-day-off approach; however, this isn't mandatory, and in any case you shouldn't overdo it. In essence, if 85%-90% of your meals are "clean" you should see good results. This 6-1 ratio is generally fine and doesn't require too much thought; however avoid pigging-out or binging excessively.
- Drink plenty of fresh clean water every day.
- Mix in some vitamin supplements and antioxidants—there's a good list of supplements in the next chapter.

GROUP A

Eat as much of these foods as you like:

- Lean beef, chicken or pork
- Whole eggs , egg yolks and egg whites
- Fish, shrimp, scallops, oysters, clams, crabs, lobsters
- Lettuce and salad greens, all varieties
- Broccoli, cabbage, cauliflower, eggplant, green beans, peas, asparagus, spinach, kale, collard greens, mushrooms, celery, bell peppers, chilies, squash, zucchini, artichokes, okra, garlic, onions, leeks, tomatoes, turnips, Brussels sprouts, Cucumbers, Avocados
- Lentils, all varieties
- Beans, all varieties, including refried beans, baked beans, bean soup
- Garbanzo beans aka chick peas, and hummus, all varieties

- Soybeans, including roasted soybeans and edamame
- Soy products, including tofu, tempeh, soy burgers, etc.
- Ice tea, coffee, club soda, herbal tea, diet soda
- High quality protein shakes and protein bars, as long as they are very low in sugar and very high in protein. Whey, soy, casein, egg and other types of protein isolates are fine. Read labels and compare; look for quality.
- Nuts (in moderation)
- Peanut butter and other nut butters (in moderation)
- Olive oil
- Butter (in moderation)
- Safflower, coconut, corn, peanut and other healthy vegetable oils

GROUP B

Avoid these foods, except during cheat meals:

- Pasta, including whole wheat pasta
- Bread, including whole wheat bread
- Rice, including brown rice
- Tortillas, including both corn and flour tortillas
- Chips, including potato chips, tortilla chips, corn and whole grain chips
- All other foods that contain flour, such as biscuits, cakes, pancakes and waffles
- Sugar, including white sugar, brown sugar, cane sugar, agave nectar, honey, corn syrup and high-fructose corn syrup
- All foods that contain sugar, including candy, sugary soda, pastries and ice cream
- Fruit and fruit juices
- All breaded deep-fried foods, including fried chicken, tempura, fish and chips, etc.
- Potatoes, including baked potatoes, mash potatoes, French fries, etc.
- Yams and sweet potatoes
- Corn on the cob
- Beets
- Carrots
- Dairy products

Always avoid hydrogenated and partially-hydrogenated oils in food, as they are *extremely* bad for you. Hydrogenated oils are among the very worst substances you can put into your body and are *not* healthy—they adversely affect your cholesterol levels and your cardiovascular health, and they may even be carcinogenic. Avoid them. Read labels. If a food item contains hydrogenated or partially hydrogenated oil—or if you even see the word "hydrogenated" anywhere in the list of ingredients—then it is *not* good for you, and you are *much* better off avoiding it. If you buy movie theater popcorn or deep-fried foods from snack bars, ask the vendor what kind of oil they use; any kind of oil is ok, really, even pure butter or lard, as long as it's not hydrogenated. You may have to have them physically show you the container of cooking oil, as many vendors, cooks and even restaurant owners don't seem to be able to read labels carefully, or to grasp the distinction between good and bad cooking oils.

Healthy casino-food meals

Here are a few super healthy casino food meals that are compatible with the Simple Poker Diet. These are just a few examples, feel free to mix and match.

- Chicken Satay, Sunomuno salad
- Denver omelet, sliced tomatoes, lima beans
- Two grilled hamburger patties, a bowl of hummus, celery
- Egg salad, mixed green salad, onion soup
- Roasted pork chops, sautéed broccoli, cabbage soup
- Baked sea bass, avocado, refried beans, sliced raw bell peppers
- Roasted chicken, green salad
- Steak, sautéed onions and mushrooms, sliced tomatoes, green salad
- One cup of almonds, two hard boiled eggs, sautéed zucchinis
- Caesar salad with grilled chicken, two hard boiled eggs
- Cobb Salad (no croutons, no cheese), vegetable beef soup
- Grilled prawns, grilled cod and roasted brocollini
- Bowl of hummus, roasted chicken, mixed green salad
- Beef skewers, refried beans, tomatoes
- Vietnamese Pho soup, with extra vegetables and no noodles
- Thai chicken curry, with Thai cucumber salad
- BBQ chicken, green beans and hummus
- Black bean chicken, with vegetable and tofu stir fry
- Prime rib, with sautéed spinach and brocolli
- Lobster, with sautéed eggplant and butternut squash
- Kobe beef strips, egg salad, mixed greens with balsamic dressing

A note on alcohol

You may have noticed that I have avoided saying anything about alcohol. I realize that some of us do drink beer, wine or liquor on occasion, perhaps frequently, and I am not going to be judgmental about it. Alcohol does contain calories however, so if you do drink just be aware that you *are* consuming extra calories, which probably will have some affect on your overall results with the Simple Poker Diet. This can be a perfectly acceptable tradeoff for many people, however it does help to be aware of it and to make some adjustments, including drinking more fresh water. Also, be aware that there is a crucial difference between hard liquors such as vodka, gin or rum, which actually contain *zero* carbohydrates, and other drinks such as beer, liqueurs and mixed cocktails, which often contain *a lot* of carbohydrates. A shot of vodka or a gin with club soda, for example, has zero grams of carbohydrate, while a tall glass of beer or a mixed drink could easily have 20-30 grams of carbohydrate or even more, and approximately the same amount of alcohol. Too many *empty* carbohydrates from drinking will tend to increase your blood glucose levels and your caloric intake, which in turn will tend to make you gain weight. Wine, on the other hand, while it does contain *some* carbohydrates, contains far less than most beers or mixed drinks. Wine also contains potent anti-oxidant compounds and nutrients, which are known to be beneficial for one's health. Wine also has a reputation for being milder, more soothing, and less harsh on your body than hard alcohol is. Keep in mind that this section *should in no way* be construed as *advising* anyone to drink alcohol. If you don't drink, great, you won't have to worry about the extra calories or any of the potentially negative effects of alcohol.

A bit of perspective on nutrition

It's generally true that many poker players eat somewhat erratically; and if you find that you're eating lots of junk food, especially at the casino or at restaurants, then you'll probably benefit quite a lot from using the Simple Poker Diet, or at least incorporating some of its broad concepts. It's easy to follow because you don't have to count calories or starve yourself, and you have many delicious and satisfying food choices; and this plan *is* firmly rooted in sound nutritional concepts. If you are currently overweight, lack muscle tone, have low energy or suffer from heartburn and indigestion, then you will see immediate improvements on the Simple Poker Diet. Merely cutting out the sugary, fatty, starchy, deep-fried and high carbohydrate foods from your diet will instantly benefit you. Of course, if you deviate from the plan or make mistakes, just try to do better at your next meal, and correct the trend. Your long-term results are what really matters.

Super supplements for poker players

Why take supplements?

In this section, we're going to look at the vitamins, herbs and other nutritional supplements that can tremendously increase your health, vitality, energy level and lifespan. These supplements can help you lower bad cholesterol, raise good cholesterol, lower the risk of cardiovascular disease, increase heart health, improve vital hormone levels, increase testosterone production, slow the aging process, lose excess weight, increase strength, increase stamina, improve mental focus and memory, and increase your chances of longevity. If you're like most people, you already take some supplements and understand their value; what's presented here is a catalogue of the most cutting edge modern supplements that can help you take it to the next level. Keep in mind that not all supplements are for all people, and that you never want to overdo it or take too much of anything. Moderation is always a good principle to adhere to regarding nutrition, *especially* when it comes to supplements. You are encouraged to continue your learning process and to do additional research; reading encyclopedia articles on the Internet and talking to the clerk at your local health food store is a good place to start if you have more questions. As always, consult your physician if you have any existing health problems before trying new supplements.

Welcome to the world of high octane

In the modern world, we are constantly exposed to pollution, stress and environmental contaminants. More and more people are trying to balance the scales by supplementing with vitamins, antioxidants, herbs, amino acids and super-nutrients; and these days, supplements are better and easier to find than ever before. Whether you are casually shopping at your local health food store or buying pure supplement powders in bulk from labs and importers on the Internet, you have unprecedented opportunity to find what you want and to get a great deal on it.

The science behind nutritional supplements is always evolving and expanding, and the availability of high quality supplements today is greater than ever. This includes exotic super-fruit and berry extracts with potent antioxidant properties, pharmaceutical grade fish oils and lipid compounds that fight bad cholesterol and inflammation, and pure amino acids that can help regenerate muscle and organ tissue and rapidly boost the health of your vascular system. A wide selection of natural herbs and extracts are available also, that boost alertness, mental focus, stamina, digestion, sexual performance and more.

Never stop learning

The reader is encouraged to do additional research regarding all of the supplements in this chapter—knowledge is power. The modern science of biology is rapidly advancing, and keeping current with new developments can give you a big advantage; while at the same time marketing-driven information about supplements can be misleading. Looking deeper into *why* certain nutrients help your body can lead to key insights and help you avoid wasting money or taking unnecessary supplements.

How to save money and get the best supplements

Ultimately, the purest form of any supplement is the best. Be aware that some retail supplements, even expensive ones, may contain only marginal amounts of the nutrient or herb you are trying to supplement. If you look around, you should be able to find access to growers, laboratories and wholesalers who can sell you pure and highly potent herbs, stacks and amino compounds at a fraction of the cost of highly marketed and processed commercial supplements. Tapping into abundant and reasonably priced sources of supplements like high quality Ginseng, Ginkgo, L-Arginine Alpha Ketoglutarate (AAKG), L-Glutamine, and fish oils will save you money and change your whole outlook on supplementing. Taking a spoonful of a key amino, or making a batch of powerful tea from raw ginseng roots can be fantastic: your body quickly assimilates it, and it's highly potent. Of course, pre-packaged pills, stacks, and energy drinks can also be great; but do some research and look around for pure sources as you gain experience.

In the following section, we're going to be looking at specific vitamins, nutrients and herbs for improving:

- Heart Health
- Weight loss and Fat Burning
- Sexual Energy and Stamina
- Resistance to Free Radicals and Environmental Stress
- Brain Power
- Digestion
- Lean Muscle Mass
- Energy Levels

Keep in mind that some supplements are listed in multiple categories. I've attempted to give a discrete list of the nutrients and herbs that are the most beneficial and targeted for each category; look for connections, think in terms of total-body health, and keep learning.

Supplements for Heart Health

What is the endothelium?

The endothelium is a layer of living cells that line the inside of all the arteries and veins in your body's cardiovascular system. The endothelium acts as a selective barrier in the blood vessel walls, and is instrumental to the body's immune system as well as nitric oxide production and the functions of vasoconstriction and vasodilation, which regulate blood pressure. With a healthy endothelium lining the walls of your circulatory system, your risk of heart attack, stroke and cardiovascular disease is extremely low. A healthy circulatory system means that your muscle and organ tissues are well oxygenated, which equates to good energy levels, stamina, sexual function, skin tone, blood pressure and health.

By contrast, a distressed, impaired and unhealthy endothelium is regarded as a hallmark of cardiovascular disease and can lead directly to heart attack and stroke. When the endothelium suffers from chronic inflammation, thickening and the fatty build up of cholesterol, lipids and minerals known as atherosclerosis, the tissues and organs of your body will receive less oxygen and your energy and concentration will be diminished; you will also be at far greater risk of heart attack, stroke, erectile dysfunction, Diabetes and even Alzheimer's disease. Smoking, chronic stress, high levels of cholesterol and lipoproteins in the blood, free radicals, chemicals, pollution, obesity, inactivity, bacterial infections and poor nutrition can injure your body's precious endothelium in a vicious cycle that, when it becomes chronic, causes the death of millions of people each year. The *primary* reason cigarette smoking increases your risk of cardiovascular disease is that cigarette smoke distresses and poisons the endothelium—even a single cigarette can have a dramatically negative effect on your body's circulatory system— stunning, poisoning and distressing the delicate inner layer of living cells within the blood vessels.

What does heart disease look like?

High levels of bad cholesterol, triglycerides, iron and low-density lipoproteins in the blood; a circulatory system damaged over time by free radicals, stress hormones, and infections... its vessels thickening with oxidized fatty buildup; impaired and deadened endothelial function; chronic high blood pressure; inflammation of organs and blood vessels; excessively high blood sugar levels; a weakened immune system. Low-density lipoproteins, cholesterol and excess minerals build up in pockets of dangerous sludge within the walls of the blood vessels, which can rupture suddenly and clog the blood supply to the heart or brain, resulting in heart attack, stroke and death. This is what cardiovascular disease looks like.

Heart health supplement list

These supplements are recommended if you'd like to:

- Lower bad cholesterol and increase good cholesterol
- Decrease excess lipoproteins in the blood
- Reduce inflammation
- Improve circulation
- Increase the body's production of nitric oxide
- Help the body to mop up and eliminate free radicals
- Decrease bacteria and fight infections
- Improve your body's electrolyte balance
- Nourish the heart and circulatory system

Multivitamin supplement	A good multivitamin covers the bases and will prevent most nutrient deficiencies.
Vitamin C	Powerful anti-oxidant; slows down cardiovascular disease; improves endothelial health; helps neutralize lipoproteins.
L-Lysine	Lowers levels of lipoproteins in the blood.
L-Proline	Lowers levels of lipoproteins in the blood.
Vitamin E (Natural, with mixed tocopherols)	Antioxidant; beneficial for arterial health; lowers risk of heart attack and stroke. Combine with CoQ10 for optimum usage.
Tocotrienols	Powerful antioxidant form of vitamin E; helps prevent oxidation of lipoproteins in bloodstream.
B-Complex Vitamins	Very beneficial for health of endothelium; calming, soothing and nourishing to the nervous system; protects from stress.
Niacin	Increases good cholesterol and lowers bad cholesterol; improves endothelial health.

Vitamin K-2	Beneficial for endothelial health; reduces arterial plaques.
Magnesium	Beneficial for cardiac metabolism and endothelial health.
Potassium	Helps in regulating heart rhythm; maintains proper muscle and nerve function; regulates fluid balance in body.
Fish Oil	Decreases inflammation; decreases triglycerides and lipoproteins; improves health of endothelium; lowers blood pressure; decreases blood viscosity; increases good cholesterol.
CLA (Conjugated Linoleic Acid)	Reduces bad cholesterol, increases good cholesterol; reduces triglycerides; reduces inflammation; reduces high blood pressure; reduces Cancer risk.
Flax Seed Oil	Lowers bad cholesterol; reduces triglycerides; reduces blood viscosity and clotting; reduces Cancer risk; improves calcium absorption.
CoQ10	Excellent antioxidant; improves function of heart cells; improves heart health; energizes heart; reduces high blood pressure; highly beneficial for brain and nervous system; anti-aging nutrient.
Nattokinase	Lowers high blood pressure; thins blood; improves circulation and prevents clots.
Lumbrokinase	Lowers high blood pressure; thins blood; improves circulation and prevents clots.
Policosanol	Lowers bad cholesterol and increases good cholesterol.

Red Yeast Rice	Reduces bad cholesterol.
D-Ribose	Good for heart muscle; increases energy.
L-Carnitine	Lowers triglycerides; beneficial for cardiac muscle and endothelium; reduces arterial plaques; increases fat burning.
L-Arginine Alpha Ketoglutarate (AAKG)	Bio-available form of L-Arginine; beneficial for the endothelium; increases the body's production of nitric oxide; increases blood flow and oxygenation; antioxidant.
L-Glutamine	Helps regenerate smooth muscle tissue, including blood vessels.
Garlic Extract (odorless)	Decreases bad cholesterol and increases good cholesterol; decreases homocysteine; increases endothelial health; increases nitric oxide production.
Green Tea Extract	Powerful antioxidant; lowers bad cholesterol; burns fat; promotes weight loss; boosts immune system.
Granulated Lecithin	Helps body metabolize, dissolve and remove fats and lipoproteins in the bloodstream; decreases bad cholesterol.
Guggal	Herb; Lowers bad cholesterol; lowers triglycerides; reduces lipoproteins in the blood.
Resveratrol	Powerful antioxidant; protects blood vessels and brain from oxidation of bad cholesterol.
Dan Shen	Herb; Reduces blood viscosity; liver tonic.

Heart health super stack

CoQ10 + vitamin C + L-Lysine + tocotrienols + B-complex + niacin + vitamin K-2 + fish oil + policosanol + L-arginine + resveratrol + granulated lecithin

Supplements for weight loss and fat burning

Losing excess weight and body fat and keeping trim is always a prime objective of health and appearance conscious people. If your body carries less fat, you'll have greater energy and stamina, you'll be sexier and look better, you'll have less soreness and joint pain, and your risk of heart disease, Cancer and Diabetes will be much lower.

Fat burning supplement list

These supplements are recommended if you'd like to:

- Increase your fat burning metabolism
- Lower your blood glucose levels
- Eliminate excess toxins from your body
- Dissolve lipoproteins in your body
- Decrease your appetite

Choline and Inositol	Helps the body metabolize lipoproteins; burns fat.
Alpha-Lipoic Acid	Reduces blood sugar levels; reduces triyglicerides; reduces bad cholesterol; helps the body burn fat and build muscle.
L-Methionine	Antioxidant; helps the body metabolize and lipoproteins and fat; helps body to excrete heavy metals.
Chromium Picolinate	Fat burner.
Green Tea Extract	Burns fat; powerful antioxidant; helps to regulate blood glucose; reduces absorption of carbohydrates; increases metabolism.
Green Tea	Burns fat; powerful antioxidant; helps to regulate blood glucose; reduces absorption of carbohydrates; increases metabolism.
Garlic Extract	Powerful antioxidant; increases fat burning and weight loss; lowers cholesterol; increases nitric oxide production.
Garcinia Cambogia	Reduces appetite; burns fat and

	slows the body's fat storage process; helps to regulate blood glucose.
Gymnema Sylvestre	Reduces blood sugar levels; reduces sugar cravings.
Cinnamon	Lowers bad cholesterol; anti-clotting effect on the blood; reduces blood sugar levels; fat burner.
Acai Berry Extract	Antioxidant; improves health of endothelium; lowers bad cholesterol; burns fat; detoxifier.
Black Tea	Antioxidant; good for the endothelium; increases metabolism; lower bad cholesterol.
Hoodia Tea	Appetite suppressant; fat burner.
Granulated lecithin	Fat burner; helps to metabolize fat; dissolves fats and lipoproteins; increases metabolism.
Caffeine	Fat burner; diuretic; increases metabolism; reduces hunger.
Ginger	Fat burner; increases metabolism.
Guggal	Lowers blood sugar levels; fat burner; helps to metabolize lipoproteins.

Fat-burning super stack

Choline and Inositol + L-Methionine + green tea extract + garlic extract + cinnamon + Alpha-Lipoic Acid

Supplements for sexual health and hormonal balance

Modern anti-aging science is increasingly discovering that preserving and restoring key hormones to the body is the essential key for preserving youth, vitality, attractiveness and sexual potency into old age. Nutrients and herbs can provide powerful tonics to your body, helping to preserve its energy and to nourish and recharge vital hormone production.

Sexual health supplement list

These supplements are recommended if you'd like to:

- Improve your body's production of nitric oxide
- Increase testosterone
- Balance your hormones
- Improve your sexual performance
- Decrease recovery time

Vitamin D-3	*The super supplement*. Highly beneficial for the body's hormonal balance; vitamin D3 is actually a hormone that is instrumental in regulating the body's metabolic processes; increases testosterone production in males; burns fat; strengthens immune system; multiple anti-aging effects.
Pumpkin Seed Oil Capsules	Improves prostate health; lowers bad cholesterol, raises good cholesterol.
Cod Liver Oil Capsules	Lowers bad cholesterol, raises good cholesterol; rich natural source of vitamin E, A and D.
American Ginseng Red Ginseng White Ginseng Korean Ginseng Chinese Ginseng	Adaptogenic herb; very healthy for the endothelium; increases nitric oxide production; helps to regulate blood pressure; helps to regulate blood sugar; powerful antioxidant; aphrodisiac properties; reduces sexual recovery time; good for recovery from strenuous workouts and

	physical exertion; replenishes adrenal glands and protects against stress; soothing and healing properties; increases oxygenation of tissues; strong anti-aging properties.
Saw Palmetto	Beneficial for the prostate gland; nourishing and anti-inflammatory properties.
L-Glutamine	L-Glutamine helps your body regenerate and repair smooth muscle tissue. Current research suggests that the health of vascular smooth muscle tissue in the reproductive system is very essential to sexual performance.
L-Arginine Ketoglutarate	Boosts nitric oxide production; boosts oxygenation of muscles and organ tissues; nourishes the endothelium.
Maca	Known as the "South American Ginseng". Adaptogenic; aphrodisiac and energizing properties; antioxidant; replenishes adrenals; beneficial for pituitary and gonads; soothing to the body; anti-inflammatory; protects body from stress; sexual rejuvenator.
Sarsaparilla	Extremely beneficial for the body's hormonal balance; boosts testosterone levels; sexual rejuvenator; soothing to the body; combats effects of stress.
Fo-Ti	Increases energy and sexual vigor; anti-aging herb.
Ashwagandha	Antioxidant; beneficial for endothelium; anti-stress; anti-microbial; aphrodisiac.
Astragalus	Beneficial for endothelial health; tonic for major organs;

	aphrodisiac properties.
Horny Goat Weed	Beneficial for endothelial health; increases blood flow; increases sexual desire and energy.
Oregano	Powerful antioxidant; especially beneficial for the prostate gland; anti-inflammatory properties; soothing for the entire body; strong anti-bacterial properties.
Tribulus Terrestris	Increases testosterone production; tonic and balancing effect on endocrine system; increases sexual desire and energy; helps to burn fat and build muscle; helps to regulate blood pressure.
Dong Quai	*[For Females Only]* Tonic effects for the female reproductive system.
Black Cohosh	*[For Females Only]* Beneficial for female reproductive system; reduces hot flashes; reduces vaginal dryness; reduces menstrual irregularities and PMS.
Wild Yam	*[For Females Only]*Helps to balance female reproductive system; reduces cramps, discomfort and other effects of PMS and menstruation.

Sex-booster super stack

Vitamin D-3 + Ginseng + Tribulus Terrestris + Sarsaparilla + L-Arginine Alpha Ketoglutarate

Supplements for fighting free radicals and preventing cell damage

Free radicals can be created in your body as a result of oxidative stress, environmental pollution, trans-fats, excess stress hormones, and chemical food additives. Free radicals can break down body tissues and damage cells, accelerating the aging process and increasing your susceptibility to Cancer, Cardiovascular Disease, dementia and other health problems. Antioxidant nutrients and herbs clean up and neutralize dangerous free radicals in your body.

Antioxidant supplement list

These supplements are recommended if you'd like to:

- Reduce free radicals in your body
- Detoxify
- Lower your risk of Cancer, dementia and heart disease
- Increase your energy level
- Protect yourself from stress
- Look better
- Live longer

Vitamin C	Powerful antioxidant.
Vitamin E	Powerful antioxidant.
Beta Carotene	Powerful antioxidant.
Grape Seed Extract	Powerful antioxidant.
Green Tea	Powerful antioxidant.
Roobois Tea (aka "Red Tea")	Powerful antioxidant.
Black Tea	Powerful antioxidant.
Resveratrol	Powerful antioxidant.
N-Acetyl-Cysteine	Powerful antioxidant.
Goji Berry Powder	Powerful antioxidant.
Acai Berry	Powerful antioxidant.
Inositol Hexaphosphate	Powerful antioxidant.
Aronia Berry Powder	Powerful antioxidant.
Maqui Berry Powder	Powerful antioxidant.
Cacao Nibs or Unsweetened Cocoa	Powerful antioxidant.
Cat's Claw	Powerful antioxidant.

Supplements for your brain

Understanding which nutrients and herbs are most beneficial and nourishing for your brain can give you a big boost in every area of your life.

Brain-booster supplement list

These supplements are recommended if you'd like to:

- Think more clearly
- Improve concentration
- Have more mental energy
- Lower your risk of Alzheimer's and dementia
- Immunize yourself from stress
- Improve your sleep

Ginkgo Biloba	Increases blood flow to brain; good for the endothelium.
Lecithin Granules or Capsules	Super brain food; replenishes neurotransmitters; boosts alertness; fights fatigue.
Choline and Inositol	Nourishes brain processes.
GABA (Gama-AminoButryc-Acid Powder)	Has beneficial effects on brain chemistry; reduces stress; natural sleep enhancer.
Melatonin	Helps synchronize biological clock; powerful brain antioxidant; induces sleep.
CoQ10	*Highly* beneficial for brain and nervous system.
L-Taurine	Beneficial for brain and nervous system; helps regulate blood pressure.
St. John's Wort	Known to reduce depression, anxiety, OCD and PMS.

Mental recharge and brain-booster super stack

Choline and Inositol + L-Glutamine + granulated lecithin + vitamin D3 + Ginkgo Biloba

Supplements for the digestive system

Indigestion, constipation and heartburn bother many people occasionally; oftentimes stress is involved in temporary flare-ups, however if these conditions become chronic they can seriously affect one's quality of life. Eating a good diet that is high in vegetables, fresh water, lean protein and complex carbohydrates, and is low in sugar, starches and rancid fats is certainly the best preventative for such GI troubles; however, certain supplements can give you an additional edge.

Digestive system supplement list:

These supplements are recommended if you'd like to:

- Improve digestion
- Reduce or eliminate heartburn
- Reduce or eliminate constipation

Probiotics	Improves digestion; decreases cholesterol; lowers Cancer risk; increases metabolism.
Kombucha Tea	Probiotic; lowers cholesterol; soothing tonic; detoxifying.
Psyllium Husks, or	Improves regularity; improves intestinal health; reduces toxicity; lowers cholesterol.
Ground Flax Seed	Improves regularity; improves intestinal health; reduces toxicity; lowers cholesterol.
Water Soluble Wheat Fiber	Improves regularity.
Barley Tea (Mugi Cha)	Soothing for digestive system; removes excess lipoproteins.
Bromelain	Enzyme helps in the digestion of proteins; aids in metabolism of lipoproteins.
Papaya Enzymes	Enzyme that aids in digestion; soothing to the system.
L-Glutamine	Nourishes the regeneration of the lining and tissues of the intestines and stomach.

Supplements for building muscle

Eating lots of high quality lean protein is the best recipe for boosting muscle mass, and adding-in protein shakes and supplements can be great. Additionally, there *are* a few amino acids and other nutrients that can be supplemented in isolation with good effects. These key nutrients can significantly decrease workout recovery times, and skyrocket energy levels and muscle development.

Muscle building supplement list

These supplements are recommended if you'd like to:

- Build muscle
- Get stronger
- Decrease recovery time after workouts
- Increase testosterone

L-Arginine AKG	Nourishes and triggers nitric oxide production, muscle oxygenation and pump.
Cod Liver Oil	In combination with vitamin D-3, increases testosterone production in males.
L-Glutamine	Decreases workout recovery time; helps the body repair muscle tissue.
L-Citrulline	Metabolizes in the body into a bio-available form of L-Arginine, which increases nitric oxide production.
L-Isoleucine	Good for muscle building and muscle recovery.
BCAA Compounds	Extra supplementation of the non-essential yet vital branch chain amino acids can significantly help your body build muscle and recover from intense workouts.

Supplements for rejuvenation and energy

Energy drinks are very popular nowadays, however many of them contain too much caffeine and sugar. All of the nutrients and herbs in this section can help boost your energy levels; many of them have been well known and treasured since ancient times for their revitalizing, soothing, tonic and energizing properties.

Energy boosting supplement list

These supplements are recommended if you'd like to:

- Increase energy
- Replenish your adrenal glands
- Fight free radicals
- Maintain focus and concentration
- Detoxification
- Balance hormones

Vitamin D-3	Super supplement; anti-aging vitamin par excellence.
CoQ10	Super supplement; taking CoQ10 has a spectrum of good effects for your entire body.
American Ginseng	Boosts energy; fights stress; replenishes hormones; adaptogenic.
Red Ginseng	Boosts energy; fights stress; replenishes hormones; adaptogenic.
Siberian Ginseng	Boosts energy; fights stress; replenishes hormones; adaptogenic.
Ginkgo Biloba	Increases blood flow to the brain; antioxidant; boosts energy.
Maca	Known as the "South American Ginseng"; energizing; adaptogenic.
Guarana (contains caffeine)	Powerful antioxidant; rich in nutrients; energizing.
Shitake Mushrooms	Whole body tonic;

	antioxidant; detoxifiying properties; lowers cholesterol.
Reishi Mushrooms	Whole body tonic; antioxidant; detoxifiying properties; lowers cholesterol.
Yerba Mate	Energizing; antioxidant; powerful anti-aging properties.
Glucosamine and Chondroitin	Strengthens and nourishes cartilage; reduces joint inflammation; reduces joint pain.
MSM (Methylsulfonylmethane)	Strengthens connective tissue and joints; reduces arthritis and inflammation.
Fo-Ti	Energizing; rejuvenating.
Green Tea Extract	Energizing; antioxidant; immune system booster; adaptogenic.
L-Taurine	Energy booster; antioxidant; beneficial for the brain.
D-Ribose	Energizing; nourishes and boosts cell metabolism and energy transfer.
L-Carnitine	Energizing; good for heart muscle.
Sarsaparilla	Tremendous natural balancer of hormones; antioxidant; soothing; energizing.

Bibliography

Alexander, Mathias and Maisel, Edward. *The Alexander Technique: The Essential Writings of F. Matthias Alexander*. Citadel, 2000.

Atlas, Charles. *Ten Steps to a Better Body: An Introduction to Fitness*. Chamberlain Bros., 2005.

Brill, Peggy and Couzens, Gerald. *The Core Program: Fifteen Minutes a Day that Can Change Your Life*. Bantam, 2003.

Caro, Mike. *Caro's Book of Poker Tells.* Cardoza, 2003.

Chow, David. *Kung Fu: History, Philosophy, and Technique*. Unique Publications, 1980.

Franklin, Eric. *Pelvic Power: Mind/Body Exercises for Strength, Flexibility, Posture, and Balance for Men and Women*. Princeton Book Company, 2003.

Gray, Henry. *Gray's Anatomy: The Classic Collector's Edition*. Garmercy, 1988.

Hanna, Thomas. *Somatics, Reawakening the Mind's Control of Movement, Flexibility and Health*. Da Capo Press, 1988.

Iyengar, B.K.S. *Light on Yoga*. George Allen and Unwin, 1965.

Ledoux, Joseph. *The Emotional Brain: The Mysterious Underpinnings of Emotional Life*. Simon and Schuster, 1998.

Maxick. *Muscle Control*. Ewart, Seymour and Co., LTD., 1911.

McKenzie, Robin. *Treat Your Own Back*. Orthopedic Physical Therapy Products, 2003.

Obeck, Victor. *Isometrics: The Static Way to Physical Fitness*. Stravon Educational Press, 1966.

O'Driscoll, Erin. *The Complete Book of Isometrics: The Anywhere, Anytime Fitness Book*. Hatherleigh Press, 2005.

Peterson, John. *Pushing Yourself to Power: The Ultimate Guide to Total Body Transformation*. Bronze Bow Publishing, 2003.

Pilates, Joseph and Robbins, Judd. *A Pilates' Primer: The Millennium Edition*. Presentation Dynamics, 2000.

Pilates, Joseph, Thomson Gordon and Robinson, Lynne. *Body Control (Using Techniques Developed by Joseph H. Pilates)*. BainBridgeBooks, 1998.

Pope, W.R. *The Science and Art of Physical Development*. London, 1902.

Sandow, Eugene. *Strength, and How to Obtain It*. Gale and Polden, LTD., 1897.

Schwarzenegger, Arnold and Dobbins, Bill. *The New Encyclopedia of Modern Bodybuilding*. Simon & Schuster, 1999.

Schwarzenegger, Arnold. *Arnold: The Education of a Bodybuilder*. Simon & Schuster, 1993.

Sears, Barry. *The Top 100 Zone Foods*. Avon, 2004.

Sinatra, Stephen; Roberts, James and Zucker, Martin. *Reverse Heart Disease Now*. Wiley, 2008.

Slansky, David and Miller, Ed. *No Limit Hold'em: Theory and Practice*. Two Plus Two Publishing LLC, 2006.

Standring, Susan. *Gray's Anatomy: The Anatomical Basis of Clinical Practice*. Churchill Livingstone, 2008.

Steward, Leighton; Bethea, Morrison; Andrews, Sam and Balart, Luis. *Sugar Busters! Cut Sugar to Trim Fat*. Ballantine Books, 1999.

Swami Svatmarama. *The Hatha Yoga Pradipika*. Forgotten Books, 2008.

Verstegen, Mark and Williams, Pete. *Core Performance: The Revolutionary Workout Program to Transform Your Body and Your Life*. Rodale Books, 2005.

Watson, Craig. *Basic Human Neuroanatomy*. Little, Brown and Company, 1991.

Whitaker, Julian. *Reversing Heart Disease*. Grand Central Publishing, 2002.

Wong, Harry. *Dynamic Strength*. Unique Publications, 1990.

Notes

Notes

Made in the USA
Monee, IL
27 September 2024

66742123R00116